Surviving *the* Waves *of*

ADHD

Surviving *the* Waves *of*
ADHD

Giving Hope and Inspiration

Nanci Beckman

Lifestyle Design, Inc.
Mission Viejo, California

Surviving *the* Waves *of* ADHD
Giving Hope and Inspiration

Nanci Beckman

Published by:
Lifestyle Design, Inc.
www.surviveADHD.com

ISBN: 978-09857763-0-5

Library of Congress Control Number: Pending

Cover and book design: Peri Poloni-Gabriel,
Knockout Design, www.knockoutbooks.com
Author Photo: Birdstudios.com
Family Portrait: CrownHeartsPhotography.com
Children's Cover photo: ValWestoverPhotography.com
Personal photos edited by: Payton Beckman

First Edition

9 8 7 6 5 4 3 2 1

Dedication

To my three Ps for having the courage and
compassion to allow me to share their very personal
and private stories in hope that we can help others
in need of some encouragement and hope in
surviving their own waves of ADHD.

To all the parents out there who are searching
for answers for their children suffering from
Attention Deficit Hyperactivity Disorder.

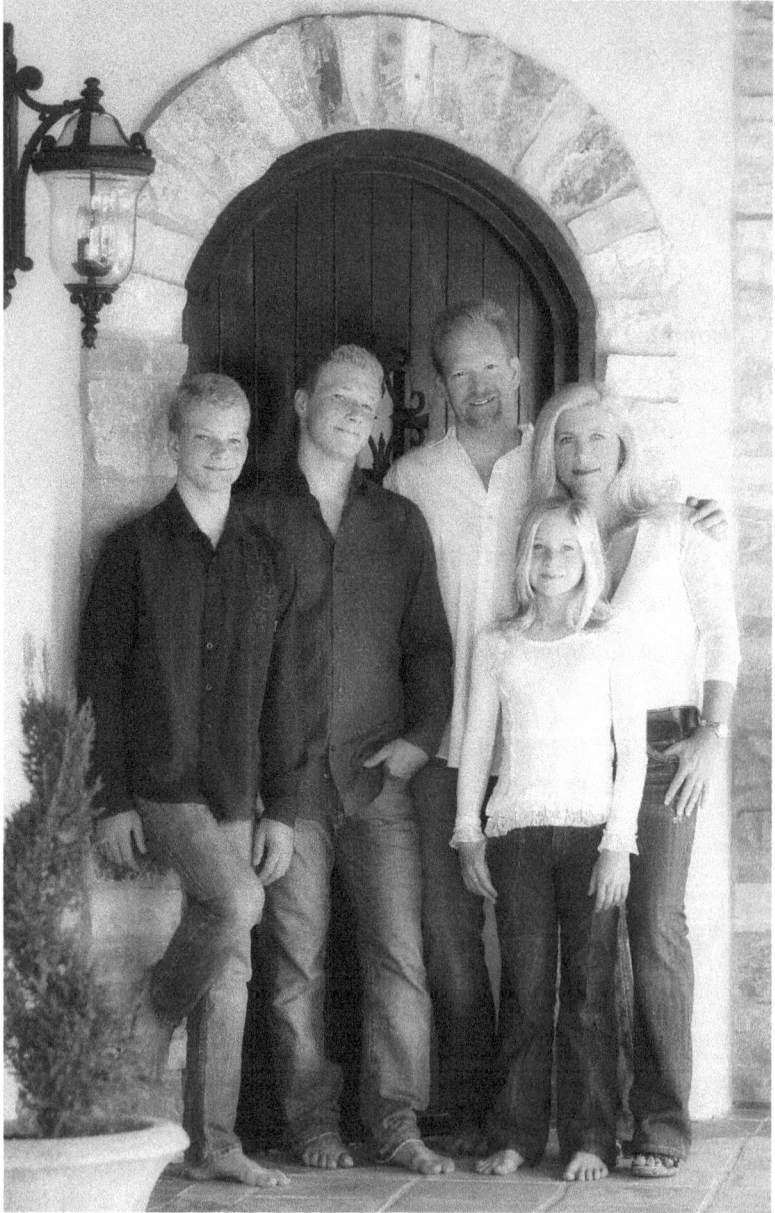

Acknowledgments

To my husband, Randy, who shares in the blessings of our three amazingly beautiful, creative, compassionate, and caring children. Thank you for our beautiful life and wonderful faith-filled journey that has guided us through our greatest challenges and greatest joys. Your having ADHD gave me a purpose in life and the passion and courage to write about it.

Portlan, you may have been my single greatest challenge in life so far, but you are worth it. You have become an incredible young man and you never cease to amaze me. Keep on writing and sharing your mind with the rest of the world.

Payton, you have always been the one I can count on to do and say the right thing. You have become a very compassionate young man, and I appreciate all your care and concern for me. Keep on drawing and shooting (photos), and please continue to share your art with the rest of the world.

Phoebe, you came into this family and made it complete with your adorable personality. You have been such a joy to parent, and your compassion and love for special needs children is mesmerizing. You light up the world with your smile and your heart, so keep spreading your gifts wherever you are and the world will be a better place.

My editor, Amy, this book would not have been published without you. I am so grateful that our paths finally crossed and we were able to use our gifts to help each other. I am so glad that you were the first person to read my story and reap the benefits from it.

Dr. Rudolf Brutoco, it is with my deepest gratitude that I say thank you to the one person who makes me feel sane. When we first met, I was drowning and you were the life preserver our family needed. Over the last twelve years you have been the genius who has kept our children feeling well throughout their many medicine changes. You have given me a wealth of knowledge and understanding into the complex world of Attention Deficit Hyperactivity Disorder. I credit you for being one of the major contributing factors for the success that our family has had with medication and learning how to survive the waves of ADHD.

Table of Contents

Testimony by the Editor

FINALLY, HERE'S A BOOK that gives parents permission to treat their child's ADHD with medication and no guilt! As a mother of a child with ADHD, I was completely against medicating my child. After spending thousands of dollars on every other natural therapy under the sun and still seeing my child struggle with homework, lose assignments, and bomb tests she knew the material for, Nanci Beckman asked me to edit her book about managing her three children and a husband with ADHD. I had read every warning against using medication, and I took on the project thinking, "I'll never medicate MY child." Yet, I was intrigued and wanted to read this book about a mom who had lived through ADHD four times and with four different cases, including her husband, and had succeeded in getting her children happy and through school. As I wasn't solving my daughter's problems I figured I could learn from Beckman's journey even if I didn't necessarily agree with her beliefs.

What can I say? She won a very skeptical me over to her side. After reading Beckman's story and meeting her successful children, I then decided that we owed it to our child to find the right doctor and at least give ADHD medications a try as a last resort. When I saw my 5th grader, who understands math well but tests very poorly, go from a D on her last math test to a score of over 100% on the next test just one week after starting her medication, I knew that medicating her was the right move.

After starting the medication, her confidence soared, her grades went up, she became more engaged in class discussions, and she could stay on topic. She actually turned in her work. She glowed at school and made more friends. Even her very messy handwriting—she suffers from dysgraphia—improved.

I got hours back into my day once she was medicated because we stopped fighting over homework. In fact, it seemed like she hardly had any homework at all after starting her medication. She could complete her work without my help or without me standing over her. My daughter did not want to take a pill at first, but after taking the medicine and feeling like she could follow along in class, stay on topic, not get bored in class, finish her work on time, and finally show her teachers how smart she really is, she now won't go to school without it.

Medication didn't solve every problem, but it has improved my daughter's life and the life of my family. Luckily she has not suffered any side effects of the stimulant medication, although we continue to keep a close eye on her growth, diet, and blood pressure. Every child is different and reacts differently to meds, but in my case, my daughter is a completely different student because I had the chance to read Beckman's book, change my views, and make the right choice for my child. I hope you too can learn from Beckman's many years' experience of surviving the waves of ADHD and find the right help for your family.

—AMY FOX, *editor and mother of a child with ADHD*

Introduction

As a mother of three children who all have different symptoms of Attention Deficit Hyperactivity Disorder (ADHD), plus being married to a man who also has ADHD, I felt compelled to share my story with parents facing similar problems. When I first realized that there was something going on with my oldest child, Portlan, I had never heard of ADHD. Not knowing how to help him, I began to experience anxiety and fear like never before. Here was an amazing boy who up to age eight I felt confident would have an incredibly easy and successful school experience from his elementary years through high school and college. But by the time Portlan was ten, I was feeling waves of shock and questioning whether he would be attending a regular high school at all. I seriously thought he would be in juvenile hall by age fifteen and certainly not allowed to drive a car! How could such an extremely bright, witty, and charming child be so troubled?

After we finally got Portlan diagnosed with ADHD and Oppositional Defiance Disorder (ODD), and then eventually into a military school for behavioral training, I realized that my second son, Payton, who was so respectful and so well disciplined was really struggling in school as well. Only he had completely different symptoms from what Portlan exhibited. At this point I was experiencing constant waves of panic and concern.

Once I got Payton diagnosed with ADHD and on his way to a more successful and happy learning experience I began to realize that my youngest child, Phoebe, was having some problems too! How could all three of my children have ADHD and yet have such different symptoms? Throughout all the testing with the children we began to realize that my husband had ADHD as well. The waves were breaking over my head by now, and some days I felt like I was going to drown.

I started writing about our chaotic journey so I would have a record of everything we had been through. The journal has evolved into this book, which I share with other parents so they can learn from my experience and begin to get their children the support they need. I wish that I had been able to read a book about a family that was struggling with all the same issues we went through and had known that there can be a successful ending. I was so terrified when I was going through the process of discovery and dealing with all the unknowns about ADHD medications, therapy, counseling, proper discipline, and finding the right doctors and books that could help me make these decisions. This is the story of how I was able to get my children diagnosed and all the struggles we went through as a family dealing with ADHD and ODD. My journey started off with learning about a disorder and has evolved into a passion and a purpose to help others.

I have spent the last twelve years talking to parents all over the country about ADHD. Whether I am in a school parking lot or waiting in lines at Disneyland, I have always been willing to discuss what I have learned through the different doctors, counselors, and my own kids with ADHD. We were extremely blessed to be able to find a really great doctor and some wonderful counselors to help us along the way. I have referred many people for help. I have had to deal with many people who disagree with my decisions and tell me that they would never medicate their children. I always tell parents who won't help their children with legal medication that their children will at some point medicate themselves, and they won't like what they choose to use!

I chose the path of medicating my children because I had tried the natural path of a strict diet with foods that were nutritious with low sugar content and had no red dye in them, along with providing the kids with high exercise and activity levels. They all took vitamins as well, and we even tried the Juice Plus gummy supplements with little to no change in focusing ability. None of my children have ever liked soda, so that was never an issue because they only drink water. They didn't even like juice, which is typically very high in sugar as well. They definitely craved the sweets but that was easy to control because I didn't buy much candy or ice cream. They are all lactose intolerant so they didn't drink milk, although they could eat cheese. Despite all this, they still needed help.

As a last result, I felt trying medication was the right thing for my kids, and I knew that I could stop the meds at any time if I felt they weren't working. There are many parents who disagree with the use of medication for ADHD, and there are many fallacies out there regarding medication. As parents we have to be advocates for our children while at the same time be realistic about possible disorders or disabilities they may have and not go into denial. We need to accept our children for who they are and embrace their uniqueness! Attention Deficit Hyperactivity Disorder is not a phase your child can grow out of. Medication may not be the right choice for some children or families, but for our family and many others I have witnessed it was the best decision we could have made for our struggling children.

Through sharing my family's stories along with the knowledge and information I have collected over the last twelve years, I wish to give you the hope and faith you'll need to survive the continuous waves of ADHD. My story has a very successful ending and I hope it will give you the strength to continue to fight for your child and not let society or the school system destroy them.

CHAPTER 1

Our First Born:
The Challenge Child!

I 'LL NEVER FORGET WHEN Portlan was born and the doctors brought him to us for the first time saying, "Here is your perfect baby boy." They had completed all the testing that they do on newborn babies, and he was normal. He was a very large baby considering my petite size and my husband being 5 feet, 10 inches tall. He weighed 9 pounds, 3 ounces, and the nurse actually screamed when he came out because of his size compared to how small I am. The doctors felt it was due to my gestational diabetes that he got so large.

Well, just like all first-time parents, we felt after four months that our baby was a genius. He could say mama and dada already and had three teeth. By eight months he had all his teeth. He was very alert and such a happy baby. He never cried, we usually had to wake him up to eat, and he slept through the night at twelve weeks old. He was as easy as it gets for a first baby. He didn't really take naps, but he was happy to entertain himself in his playpen for two hours at a time. That usually gave me a nice break.

Portlan didn't start walking until fourteen months, but that was probably due to the fact that he was still in the playpen. Once I folded that up and put it away he started walking immediately. Once he could walk, my life as I knew it was over. He was very fast and I could not take my eyes off of him for a second. By eighteen months old, he was speaking eight-word sentences and could tell me how to drive to my sister's house. He had memorized the names of all the animals in his alphabet animal book. This was not an ordinary book; the animals names were much more difficult. There was a narwhal whale, orangutang, and unicorn fish, to give a few examples. I read him the formal names expecting him to remember the simple names, but he memorized the full name of each animal.

By the time he was eighteen months he had been starting to show signs of being very strong willed. My happy, very easy baby was turning into a challenging toddler. He was so smart it sometimes scared me, and I could not get through to him if I needed him to stop doing something bad. Our biggest face-off each day was over the television buttons. Our TV sat very low to the ground, so he could easily reach it. He loved to sit and turn it on and off. I could not get him to stop no matter how many times I scolded him, and every form of punishment I used made him laugh. I thought I was going crazy that a toddler could outwit me.

Then I bought a book called *The Strong-Willed Child* to regain my ability to deal with my child. It was a great book and talked about the best way to handle a child like mine. The book explained that you needed to keep on the child no matter how many times it took and not to give up. It also explained that you should change the form of punishment each day to mix it up. I felt revitalized after reading this book and was confident that I had the tools to get through to Portlan. The next day when he started in with the TV control I walked up to him and pulled him down onto his bottom quickly and then told him NO very firmly. Well, I proceeded to do this about fifty more times before I couldn't take it any more. Portlan after about the third time thought it was fun and he loved getting all my attention. I tried to follow what the book said and changed the punishment each day, but this child had nerves of steel and super-human powers when it came to outlasting me, a twenty-seven-year-old mom with a college degree.

Portlan Starts Kindergarten

I started Portlan in kindergarten at age five. Since he has a July birthday, he was young compared to the other children in the class even though the cut-off was in December. I didn't know that most people in our area were holding back boys with summer and fall birthdays because of maturity. His social skills at that age were very advanced for a boy, so I didn't feel bad about starting him right when he turned five, and he was handling school just fine.

He was in a private school and the curriculum there was quite advanced. They were already teaching them to read, and they were taking spelling tests. Portlan was ambidextrous, so he was still trying to write with both hands. The teacher told him he had to choose, so he decided to use his right hand. I don't remember him learning to read; he could just do it. The spelling tests were a breeze and he even entered a spelling bee. He had an incredible memory, which we already knew.

For first grade we switched him to a different private school. He breezed through that year because the curriculum wasn't as advanced and was repetitive for him. He was still doing fine with the academics, but I started to notice he was having some social issues. He didn't seem to have a lot of friends and he would say, "nobody likes me," or "I don't have any friends." Now at first I thought he was just trying to get attention because he was so outgoing and social. Being a biased mom, I couldn't believe he would have trouble making friends. How was this blond-haired, blue-eyed adorable kid who could have been on a cereal box not able to find kids to play with him?

I also started noticing that he had a real compulsiveness to lie about the simplest things. He would automatically tell a lie instead of the truth. If you asked him if he brushed his teeth, his first reaction was to lie. For a while I told him I would pay him a quarter every time he told me the truth first to break this bad habit. I also noticed that he could not do his homework by himself. I had to sit with him and watch him do it or he would get up and walk away.

The final observation that really bothered me was that he would constantly interrupt people when they were talking. It didn't matter who it was: a grandparent, teacher, principal of the school, or coaches. He constantly interrupted his dad and me. He was very active and always had been, but I attributed that to being a boy. My sister and her husband always felt that my boys were really hyper, but their daughter was unusually quiet. My dad grew up with three brothers and told me that boys are busy so I brushed it off.

Then one day I was talking to a mom, and the term ADHD came up. I asked her what that was, and she explained to me that it was this disorder that some kids have. I asked her how you know if your kid has it. She said that there is a list of ten characteristics and if your child has at least four or five of them then they probably have it. But she didn't really know all of them, and she knew Portlan and said there was no way he had it. But I continued to think about this ADHD and wanted to know more about it. As I was talking to more parents about it I would gather some of the characteristics from different people. Some told me that they tend to be very hyperactive, have a hard time learning to read, they have learning disabilities, and they constantly get into trouble at school because of discipline and control issues.

By second grade Portlan's social issues were about the same. I mentioned to his new teacher some of my concerns and she told me she would keep an eye on him. When conference time rolled around she told me that she felt he was a normal boy and would grow out of his compulsive actions and interruptions in class.

Then in third grade we moved Portlan to another private school affiliated with our church and where some of his friends also went. We had hoped that he would stay there through eighth grade. He had a pretty good third grade year with a teacher who really appreciated his wit and humor. He was making more friends at this school, although they were mostly girls. Portlan was also very involved with baseball by now in the city league. He was a very good player, but he had some emotional issues on the field that were difficult to deal with. His dad and I coached most of his teams and so part of the problem was us coaching our own child. We did start to notice that he was becoming more physical and seemed to get into arguments with other boys more frequently. When we were at parties if there was a commotion going on he was usually in the middle of it. He was also getting into a lot of fights with the neighborhood kids, who were his closest friends.

A Turning Point!

As Portlan started fourth grade he was becoming more and more self-destructive. We were spending much of our time arguing with him because of his lying and sudden urge to tease his brother, incessantly. Every situation that involved a scuffle, he lied about who started it and what happened. If something was missing in the house we all knew who took it, but no matter what form of punishment we used he would not fess up. My husband and I began to argue a lot over how to handle him, and it seemed as if my other two children became nonexistent. We were spending every minute of each day dealing with Portlan. He still could not do his homework on his own, yet he aced all his tests.

Then someone recommended another book to me called, *The Wonder of Boys*, by Michael Gurian. I started reading this book and I began to learn more about boys than I ever could have learned in a biology class. This book talks about the physiological, psychological, and emotional differences between boys and girls. It also talks about how differently girls and boys are treated in school by teachers and other people in the community. The boys basically get the short end of the stick is what that portion of the book was explaining.

While I was reading this book, things continued to get worse with Portlan. His lying was at an all-time high, he was starting to steal, and his grades started plummeting for the first time. We also noticed that his self-esteem and confidence were taking a dive. Then his teacher called me one day and told me that things were disappearing in the classroom. They weren't major things just pencils, erasers, and other children's lost items.

At about the same time at home, I was missing $20 out of my wallet one night when I went to a meeting. When I got home I asked Portlan if he took it when he went to get ice cream with a friend. He told me no that he didn't need any money because his friend's mom paid. I knew that I had an extra $20 in my wallet and it crushed me to think that he would lie to me like that. My husband wanted to use his way of getting the truth out of him, but it was never very effective and I could see we were driving him away from us. So I told my husband that I would get the truth out of him but it might take a few days. I also noticed that Portlan had a new package of Pokémon cards that I had not purchased for him. Each day I questioned him about the money, and he would sit and help me try to figure out who took it. He would hug me and say, "Mom I would never steal money from you," and then give me a big kiss. That weekend my husband and I told him to go in and talk to the priest about what had happened and pray for the truth to come out. Well by the end of that week I was certain he took the money, but I needed to get him to confess to it. When we were driving home from school that Friday I asked him one more time to tell me if he stole the money. But before he answered I told him that I was going to call the mom who took him to get ice cream and ask her if he had money on him. He still showed no sign of nervousness and told me to go ahead and call her. Then I told him that I better not hear the truth from her, that if he did take the money I better hear it from him. If he did not tell me himself, his punishment would be much more severe. With that he kind of got quiet and then asked me what was going to happen to him if he did take the money.

I took the three kids to Ballpark Pizza so I could give Payton and Phoebe money to go play games while I did an interrogation on their brother. When we got to the pizza place and were alone I asked him one last time if he stole my money. He finally told me yes, and suddenly I broke down crying. He kind of panicked and asked me why I was crying. I told him that I was very concerned about his behavior and scared because I didn't know what to do for him. He explained to me that he knew it was wrong to take the money, but he just couldn't help it. There was something in his head that would make him do things he knew he shouldn't do, but he couldn't stop himself. This is the impulsivity of ADHD that kids have a very hard time controlling on their own. When we got home I called my husband at work and told him that I finally got the truth out of him and that he did take the money. He was as devastated as I was. I didn't know what else to do so I sat down and started reading my book about the wonder of boys.

I opened my book, and when I turned the page the next chapter was titled, Attention Deficit Hyperactivity Disorder. I couldn't believe it because I really wanted to know more about this disorder, ADHD. As I began to read I realized this was describing my child and that he had many of the symptoms of

ADHD. The book described children with ADHD as being typically very bright, charming, and witty, with a tendency to suffer
from compulsive lying, sneaking, and stealing, which can lead
to drug and alcohol abuse if not diagnosed. Kids with ADHD
can suffer from learning disabilities and dyslexia as well.

Medication is recommended in some cases to help the children. They basically have no pause button--if they think it they
say it or do it. Well I couldn't believe my eyes when I read
that paragraph because it described Portlan exactly. If I didn't
know better I would have thought that someone was writing
a description of my son except for the dyslexia and learning
disabilities.

I called my husband at work immediately and made him listen
while I read the definition of ADHD to him. He was shocked as I
began to read a perfect description of our child and his behavior.
He had told me once before that we could not use medication
to control our children's behavior, but at this moment I told my
husband that I am the mother and I will do what is right for
our children, even if it means giving them medication. For some
reason, and I am not sure what it is, out of most of the parents I
have counseled over the last eleven years, it's the fathers who are
very against medication for no other reason than they do not like
the idea of their child having to take a pill every day.

A Diagnosis

It was the spring of Portlan's fourth-grade year and he was nine years old. I went through our insurance to try and find a psychiatrist who could help diagnose and treat the ADHD. We had an HMO at the time, and unfortunately they referred me to a psychiatrist who wasn't specifically for kids. He did however prescribe some Ritalin (methylphenidate HCl) for Portlan. The office was not what I would call kid friendly. The psychiatrist gave me the prescription and told me to come back in six months. I couldn't believe that he didn't want to do more thorough testing and that he would prescribe a drug like Ritalin and then tell me to come back in six months. After a few months of Portlan being on the Ritalin I looked for another psychiatrist who had more experience with ADHD and children. I did find another doctor who seemed to be a little more thorough, but he gave me the same medication and had me check back in three months.

The Ritalin had definitely settled Portlan down, but he was starting to develop some nervous tics (twitches) while on the medication. His fifth-grade year was going pretty smoothly, but it helped that he had a wonderful teacher who really enjoyed his quirky sense of humor. She also happened to favor the boys over the girls, which was a nice change.

In the winter of his fifth-grade year I had a minor surgery and was as stressed out as one can get and still function. I wasn't sleeping, I couldn't eat, and I was so worried about Portlan that I was beginning to have anxiety attacks. I dragged myself to a school function one day because something was compelling me to go. While I was there I started talking to another mother, and we got on the subject of ADHD. It turned out that her children had it and she was using a doctor who specialized in working with children who have ADHD. She gave me his name and number and suggested that I call him because he had really helped her family. She warned me that he was very expensive and did not accept any insurance. I was so excited for the first time in months because I felt that I was going to be able to find help for Portlan. I was a little worried about the money, but at this point I just wanted a doctor who was kid friendly and really knew how to treat ADHD.

I called this doctor immediately and found out that it was going to be a month before I could get in. In the meantime, we were able to begin some routine testing to really get a true diagnosis for Portlan. I still had parents telling me that he did not have ADHD and that he is just really smart and probably bored in school. There are so many reasons to ignore what your children might really have because you don't want to face the truth. As a mother who has taken her career, or calling in life, as a "stay at home mom" very seriously, I was not about to take any chances and assume that my son would just outgrow these behaviors. I had put too much time and effort into this child, and even though he was my first I was not going to use that as an excuse to make any mistakes. I felt it was my job to find out as much information as I could and make sure that my child received the proper treatment.

We had some routine tests taken for Portlan. The Connors' Parent Rating scale test and the Connors' Teacher Rating scale test were some of the first. These scales rate the child's moods and activity throughout the day. The parents and teacher fill out forms and essentially rate the child on the same questions to see if he or she acts differently at home and at school. It can be very effective and gives you a relatively quick diagnosis.

After those tests confirmed that Portlan did in fact have ADHD we had more testing done. These tests can be very beneficial to diagnosing your child with ADHD: Wechsler Intelligence Scale for Children–Fourth Edition (WISC- IV), Wechsler Individual Achievement Test-Second Edition (WIAT-II), Guide to the Assessment of Test Session Behavior (GATSB), and the Bender Gestalt Test-Second Edition (BGT-II). Checklists: Behavioral Assessment System for Children, Second Edition (BASC-2), Connors-Wells' Self Report Scale (CWSRS); Multidimentional Anxiety Scale for Children (MASC). Please refer to the sidebar on Testing and Results in Chapter 2 for further explanation of these tests.

When we first met with the ADHD specialist, Dr. B, an MD with an MPH, my husband and I had a two-hour consultation with him without Portlan present. He wanted to know everything about Portlan from pregnancy on and he also wanted to know about our parents and siblings, since ADHD is very hereditary and is typically passed on to each generation. The subject turned to my husband's history. My husband has always had time issues since I have known him. He starts twenty projects and doesn't completely finish them in a timely manner. He can also have a hard time making decisions. All of these can be symptoms of ADHD. What stumped me is that he did really well in school, and one major red flag with ADHD is struggling with school. It came up that my husband chewed tobacco in high school and college. As my husband thought about the times he chewed, he realized it usually was before a big test or during finals. He chewed during his most stressful times in school and when he really needed to settle down and study.

The doctor explained to us that nicotine is a drug that can calm people down and that it definitely helps people focus. It works a lot like Ritalin (methylphenidate) except that tobacco is addictive and can lead to cancer and death. He wanted us to have Portlan stop taking the Ritalin he had been prescribed so he could see what he was really like off the medication.

The doctor recommended that we see a psychologist as well. She was a counselor who had two children of her own with ADHD. She helped us learn to deal with Portlan much better and not to engage with him. He was diagnosed with Oppositional Defiant Disorder (ODD) as well as ADHD. Children with ODD are very combative and turn every single thing in life into a fight. That was probably the hardest thing to deal with in our household. The psychologist taught us how to ignore a lot of Portlan's behavior and not be so easily drawn into his traps. Portlan's main goal was to start an argument and upset a parent. I immediately backed off and could see what the psychologist was talking about not engaging. I also stopped asking Portlan questions that I already knew the answers to and that set him up to lie. I used to ask him if he brushed his teeth, made his bed, cleaned his room, did his homework, etc. Instead of asking him if he did these things I would tell him to do it, and if he replied that he already did it then I would go and check. What was so interesting to me was that no matter how many times he lied about things, I always caught him and yet he never gave up.

In many situations, ADHD will be diagnosed along with other disorders. Check the bibliography for more great reference books that can help you to discover other childhood disorders. You might think your child has ADHD and they actually have something totally different. I read the book, *The Out-of-Sync Child*, written by a teacher, thinking that was going to be Portlan, but it completely described my sister's daughter. She read the book and realized that her daughter was suffering from Sensory Integration Disorder, which neither one of us had ever heard of before. She was able to go back to her pediatrician and get a referral to the appropriate doctor for this type of disorder.

A Better Medication

The doctor definitely wanted to start some medication with Portlan once we got all the tests back. We started with 18 mg of Concerta (methylphenidate HCI), which was a longer-lasting drug and didn't have the short-term effects of Ritalin. Within a week of him being off the Ritalin the tics subsided. Once the Concerta got into his system (about two days) we noticed a difference in him almost immediately. He was definitely calmer and not as interruptive when sitting with adults. We were at a family party, and Portlan was sitting at the table without interrupting anyone. My mother-in-law was so impressed and mentioned to my husband and me that Portlan is starting to mature because she had never seen him sit that quietly before. We looked at each other, grinned, and explained to her that he was taking medication for ADHD.

In the beginning, Portlan responded pretty well to the Concerta. He pitched the game of his life in baseball because he was able to keep his concentration while he pitched an entire eight innings. We began to sigh a little bit because things seemed to be calming down a lot around the house too. As he continued to take the medication though, we noticed that his temper seemed to flare up, and his already intense personality seemed to get more intensified. He was really bothered by the fact that he had to take medication and that that made him different from all the other kids. We ended up having to add another drug, called Zoloft (sertraline HCl), which helped to even his mood and take the edge off his angry temper. This helped him to settle down quite a bit, and he finished fifth grade pretty successfully.

For parents who are so concerned about trying out medication for their children here is something important to know: drugs like Adderall (amphetamine, dextroamphetamine), Ritalin, and Concerta (methylphenidate HCl) are quick-release drugs that get through your child's system very quickly. They are in and out, which means they do not have any long-lasting effect on them. This is why I was always willing to at least try them with my kids because if I didn't like what they were doing I could stop them immediately. Believe me, it is worth trying them for the sake of saving a child's self-confidence and even self-worth. Every child wants to do well in school. Even though some kids try to act like they don't really care that they are doing poorly in school, they do care! These medications can give your child the focusing ability that doesn't come naturally to them and help them to do better in school.

Stimulant medication can have some side effects such as nervous tics or twitches, loss of appetite, difficulty sleeping, and in some cases a child can have the reverse effect in which the stimulant actually makes the child tired. Most of these side effects are very minor and will go away once the child stops the medication. You can ask your doctor to perform an electrocardiogram (EKG) before having your child start taking the medication to rule out any undiagnosed heart problems. A complete blood panel work-up is a good idea as well to check your child's liver function. Urine tests done frequently are useful to catch if there are any underlying issues. Dr. B checks about every two months to make sure the medications are clearing the child's system and orders another follow-up blood panel six to nine months after starting the medications. Often most psychiatrists and general practitioners will not order routine tests. Only a specialist will typically request all these tests.

Portlan Starts Middle School

We had hoped that sixth grade would be a great year for Portlan. He seemed to have a really supportive homeroom teacher, and Dr. B told us it would help Portlan to be changing classes often. As usual he always started each year off with outstanding grades and the teachers all loving him. After six to eight weeks into the school year he began to slack off on his homework and the teachers got to see more of his real personality come out.

Dr. B had recommended that we switch Portlan into public school since there are a lot more kids to choose from for friends. Portlan always had a hard time fitting in with the ninety kids in his private school class. I didn't switch him yet because I was just too afraid that he would look for the worst kids on campus and become friends with them. Ever since he was two years old in preschool he was always drawn toward the one or two kids that you really wouldn't want your child to befriend. In a private school I always felt that the worst kid he could find wouldn't be so bad. Boy was I wrong about my decision to keep him in private school.

Portlan's ODD seemed to worsen as he got older and it was at an all-time high by the middle of sixth grade. His lying seemed to be getting really bad again too. Our doctor started adding in some more medication to knock his ego down since Portlan did not recognize or respect authority at all. He was given a drug called Depakote (divalproex sodium), which is an anti-seizure medication. This drug is very effective with kids like Portlan who think they are above all their peers, parents, or teachers and try to dominate every conversation. We were trying to take Portlan down a tone so that he might be able to interact more effectively with his peers. I have to admit that this drug scared me to death, but I trusted my doctor.

Portlan was taking quite a cocktail of medications by this point. I was concerned, but each time we made medication changes he would settle down and do much better for a while. I am sure that parents who are against medicating are horrified right now with all the medications we have allowed our son to take. Please keep reading because I think you will be impressed with the end of this story. At this point we were starting to threaten him with military school, since we knew he needed more discipline. We did some research and found that there was an all-boys catholic military school within twenty miles of our home. He was able to manipulate just about everyone around him, and he was so disrespectful to his teachers and other adult figures in his life that we felt that this type of school might be what he needed to change his attitude and teach him how to respect authority.

In the spring we had a meeting with all of his teachers and brought Dr. B in to speak to all of them about Portlan. I was so tired of the complaining from all of them, and they would not cut him any slack. We started the meeting with each teacher expressing his or her difficulties with Portlan. One complained that he raised his hand in class too much and wanted to answer every question. Another complained that he was always writing on something during her class. Another threw a paper Portlan had written on the table and said she couldn't believe the "crap" that he turned in. His homeroom teacher was really worried about all the medication he was on. I was always very upfront with the teachers about all the medications he was taking.

Once they all were done having their say, Dr. B explained to all of them that Portlan's prognosis was very good and that they didn't need to be so concerned about him. He told them what they needed to do was relax with him and give him some slack. So he raised his hand all the time--that was because he is hyper and by raising his hand he is moving around. The doctor told that teacher to just let him know that you can't call on him every time, but that it doesn't hurt for him to raise his hand.

He explained to the English teacher that because of the ADHD, writing papers were more difficult for him. He could think of what to write, but he lost a lot in translation while he was writing. He suggested we put a microphone on our computer so Portlan could talk his papers and suggested to the teacher that maybe Portlan could do some of his papers orally, since he loved to be in the front of the class getting attention. Dr. B gave each teacher constructive ways to deal with Portlan and stay positive with him. My husband and I left that meeting feeling so much better about Portlan and the rest of the school year.

However, I was becoming very concerned about Portlan being on so much medication. The Depakote really concerned me because that was a more-involved drug than the other medications he was taking. I spoke with Dr. B and expressed how concerned I was that Portlan was on the Depakote. We decided to back him off this drug, but I explained to the homeroom teacher that I would need her help and cooperation, plus her feedback as to how he reacted at school. She expressed her own concerns with him being on so much medication to me as well. Portlan's conduct grade at this point was a B, and he managed to be staying under the radar for discipline issues.

Within three days of him being off of the medication I received a phone call from his teacher. She was very upset and said to me, "I don't know what he was taking but please have him start taking it again." He was out of control and difficult to handle at school. I kind of chuckled and told her that I was thinking of taking him off all his meds so she could really experience the "Full Portlan." She said, "No, no, Mrs. Beckman, please don't take him off any more medication." I thought it was interesting how fast she changed from her concern with him being on so much medication to wanting to keep him on everything. We let him stay off the Depakote for about a week, but then we tried another drug called Trileptal (oxcarbazepine), which is similar to Depakote, but he did not accept this drug as well as he did the Depakote. We put him back on Depakote because he was unbearable to be around.

Portlan somehow made it through to the end of sixth grade, but not without some fireworks. In June, my husband and I were going to Hawaii for our fifteenth anniversary. The entire school year, Portlan had begged us to buy him a Palm Pilot so he could be more organized with his homework and dates of tests. He also told us that most of the kids at school had one. Of course we told him that he didn't need one and he could use the planner he already had. The day before we were to leave for Hawaii my husband went to leave for work and there was a package on our front porch. It was addressed to my husband and his company name. My husband opened the box and inside was a $600 Palm Pilot with a cover and a game. I was at the market getting all the food for the kids for the week when my husband called me. He was really upset and asked me why I ordered myself a $600 Palm Pilot. I of course had no idea what he was talking about and we both began to realize that Portlan must have ordered it over the Internet. He had hoped that it would come while we were in Hawaii and he somehow thought we would never see the charge show up on our credit card. This boy had nerves of steel and was too smart for his own good.

When I picked up all the kids from school I calmly explained that they would not be going to their uncle's house like we planned because something very serious happened at our house. The kids were all upset over what could have happened, and then I explained to them that someone had committed computer fraud in our house. I told them that I had been talking to the police about it and trying to figure out who would have done it. I told them that you can go to jail for that because it is a very serious crime. I watched Portlan through my rearview mirror the whole time and the kid didn't even flinch.

Later that evening my husband and I sat Portlan down and grilled him for two hours before we finally broke him down and got him to tell us what he did. He said he knew it was wrong the minute he did it but he couldn't control himself. We were going to cancel our trip but the doctor told us not to because then he wins again. His punishment was working all summer to raise the money for the Palm Pilot and then not get it. We wanted him to feel how hard it was to make that much money since all he did was take numbers off a credit card and type them into a computer. He needed to realize how much money he stole.

The finale to this sixth-grade year was when I received Portlan's report card two weeks into summer and he ended up getting an F in conduct. I immediately asked Portlan if anything really bad happened at school between the progress report and school getting out and he said no. So I called the school and spoke with the principal asking for an explanation as to the F Portlan got in Conduct since I had been given no warning. Six weeks before school got out he still had a B on his progress report. She didn't know why and told me she would contact his teacher. About a week later his teacher called me and when I asked her what happened she told me that he was so bad during that time he went off his meds. I explained to her that she was aware that he was off medication partially due to her concerns as well as mine. I didn't think it was fair to count that against him when it wasn't his fault that we decided to do a drastic medication change in the middle of the semester. She went on to tell me that even when he got back on his medication he never really got much better and so he deserved the F. This was just one more giant wave breaking over my head, when it came to dealing with this child in a school setting.

Military School Here We Come

I mentioned that we had been threatening military school to Portlan throughout the year. Well it was time to follow through! We contacted the school, met with the principal, toured the school, and got very excited. Next we brought Portlan to meet the principal and tour the school. While he didn't really want to attend an all-boys school, he knew it would be a good place for him. His closest friends had been girls, and it was going to be difficult for him to have no girls around. The school had the option to be a boarding school, but the nuns recommended driving him if we could handle him at home.

That summer Portlan and his brother Payton both attended summer school at the military school together to get a feel for it. Payton had asked us if he should go with Portlan because he was so concerned about him. We explained that this would be good for Portlan and that he would be fine.

When school started in the fall my husband drove Portlan to school every morning on his way to work. Then my husband would run over and pick him up at 3:00 pm and bring him back to his office. They stayed there until about 6:00 pm. Portlan was to do all his homework before he came home. This new schedule completely changed my life in the afternoons. I was actually able to help Payton and Phoebe with their homework and not chase Portlan around trying to weed through his manipulation of lies.

In the beginning, Portlan took a real "I don't care" attitude. He had to wear a full military uniform including a hat. Every morning at roll call if a student was missing any part of his uniform he received a demerit. This was a real learning experience because this kid could care less about brushing his teeth and hair before school let alone taking responsibility for being dressed in a complete military uniform. At the military school the students are given conduct cords that hang on their shoulders. If someone doesn't have his cord it is because he lost it due to an infraction. Every other Friday the boys can earn merit awards (colored bars)--just like in the real service--that go on their bar, which is pinned to their uniform and leads to an advancement in rank letting everyone know what the boy has earned. But the student must have his conduct cord in order to receive a merit award. Well finally a Friday came when Portlan should have earned a bar, but he had lost his conduct cord due to an infraction, so he wasn't able to receive it. Amazingly, this really started to bother him so after waiting the required two weeks without an infraction, he got his conduct cord back and he really tried to keep it so he could start receiving the merit awards that he earned.

The retired military officer who was in charge of disciplining the boys at the school liked Portlan a lot and always took the time to talk to him about how he could improve his behavior. I give a lot of credit to this program because it really does reach these hard-to-discipline kids. The teachers at this school were incredible too, because they were all long-time veteran teachers who didn't take any "crap" from these kids. Between the military-style discipline and the zero-tolerance teachers, Portlan was really starting to turn a corner. He was not getting into our faces nearly as much as he used to, and he wasn't so manipulative.

We told him that if he got good grades and changed his attitude by the end of seventh grade, he could maybe go back to his other school for eight grade and graduate with his friends. Well he did what he needed to do, so we did let him go back to his previous school for eighth grade. But it's probably not a decision I would make again. He had an okay year, but it would have been better if we had had him finish up at the military school.

Should Portlan Start High School?

After eighth grade, Portlan was still immature and small for his age. Most of the girls in his class were a full year older than him and the boys one to two years older. I had a really bad feeling about sending him off to high school, and I didn't know what to do. My husband had the same gut feeling that he could use an extra year. We decided to talk to Portlan and see how he felt about starting high school. He definitely didn't want to attend the private high school that we had enrolled him in, and we were still terrified at the idea of public school.

Four of Portlan's neighborhood buddies were his age but had been held back, so they were all going into eighth grade. He asked us if he could go to the public junior high and attend eighth grade there with all his friends in the neighborhood with whom he had never been in school. Plus none of the kids there would know that he was repeating eighth grade. It was kind of a win-win situation as long as he didn't get into any trouble. Dr. B kept telling me that when he got there he would quickly figure out who the good kids and bad kids were, and he would choose somewhere in the middle.

Well before summer got started we decided to make another medication change. There were some new drugs out that he could take, and we could back him off a few others. One particular drug was called Abilify (aripiprazole). So we started that, but within a week we realized that this new drug wasn't going to work for him. It was very strong and took away his whole personality. My doctor decided that since it was summer and he had been on medication for basically four years, he should take a break and let's see how he is. I was really nervous because the last time that we did this it was a disaster.

We had him stop taking all his medications, and we watched him go through a change. The new medication he had been on was very strong, so it took almost two weeks for him to get back to his usual talkative self. Even then I was concerned because he was very reserved and really calm. I had him stay with me all the time because some of the medication he had been on was really strong and a lot more concerning than Ritalin or Concerta. Over the course of maybe three to four weeks a new Portlan evolved and to this day I don't know if it was maturity, a decision to really change, or a true miracle. Portlan was a totally different kid. He was getting along with his brother and sister, and he was getting along with the neighborhood kids better too. He was very excited to be attending the public junior high that fall, and we had a really good summer. Portlan was only medicated from the age of ten until he was fourteen.

When September rolled around and he started school Dr. B wanted him to stay off medication to see how he could do academically. He told me to keep Portlan off the meds, even if he starts to get into trouble, and just see how he does. Well he got through the first semester with four A's and one B, and all the teachers there loved him. I told some of them that he had ADHD and they didn't believe me. Portlan told us how the teachers there were so much better with junior high kids than his old private school. Like his doctor told me, he immediately figured out who the wrong kids were and he didn't want anything to do with them. Because the school was so big he met a lot of different kids and if one group wasn't treating him right on a certain day then he would go hang out with a different group.

He finished his eighth grade year on the Principal's Honor Roll, and he had grown 6 inches and gained about 30 pounds. Stimulant medication can inhibit growth, but that was not true with my kids because my younger son, Payton (now in college), has not been off his meds since fourth grade and is taller than Portlan. My husband was a late bloomer and kept growing until he was twenty-two. The Ritalin and Concerta definitely contribute to weight loss since the kids have no appetite. I gave my boys protein shakes to help them gain weight.

Portlan's confidence was back and he was much more mature and ready to start high school. Someone once told me that they had never met anyone who was sorry they held a child back. They only knew people who were sorry they didn't hold a child back. This was one of the best decisions we ever made with Portlan. We were very fortunate to have the option for him to attend the public school, giving him a fresh start while repeating eighth grade.

High School and Then off to College

Portlan started high school with a mature attitude and joined the wrestling team. This sport was appropriate for him because he could put his bad temper to good use. He liked being on a team and loved the whole high school atmosphere. He continued to do well in school without the help of medication, and I prayed that he could stay focused. By his junior year he was getting tired of wrestling, so I made him try tennis. You have to understand that this kid was and still is a phenomenal athlete, but because of the ADHD he tires of things fast and gets bored. Through the course of his high school years he managed to try pole vaulting and surfing as well. He actually became a pretty good surfer and earned a varsity letter in surfing his senior year. He took some AP classes in English, since he is a brilliant writer, and someday I hope he writes a book. His poetry and vocabulary are fantastic!

Probably the single best thing he did in high school was to become very involved with the church youth group his freshman year, and that is where he found his best friends. He was able to have the good judgment to become friends with some of the smartest kids in his class, which helped to push him academically. These kids were also a really good influence on him personally. Portlan helped many kids through that church by sharing his troubling years with them through the testimonies he gave. He would talk to many kids about how out of control he was and how thankful he was to have parents who cared enough to help him. He headed up several youth activities and went on many mission trips to Mexico. His most profound mission trip was when he traveled to Rwanda with thirty other students and Pastor Rick Warren. He actually wrote and preached a sermon while he was there, and he fell in love with the people of Rwanda.

Portlan got through high school as a perfectly well-adjusted teenager and to whom I refer as my miracle child. He found his calling to help the people around him. He focused in on a private Christian college in San Diego, California, and made sure that he had his grades and SAT scores where he needed them to be so he could be successfully accepted to the school through early application. Portlan was able to stay on top of his homework and tests all through high school on his own. I did not get involved with his day-to-day schoolwork ever again after that military school!

Someone once told me that once a person starts taking medication for ADHD they can never stop. Well Portlan is proof of how false a statement that is. He has successfully "graduated from his meds," as Dr. B likes to say, and completed four years of high school and three years of college without medication. Certain phases of life may warrant a restart but that shouldn't be considered a failure! Portlan admits to sometimes having a hard time focusing, and during his second year of college he did try to use the Daytrana (methylphenidate) patches for a few months. He didn't feel that the patches made a big enough difference in his study habits to continue using them, so he stopped. He entered his junior year of college as a writing major and has still been able to cope without any ADHD meds. That may change before he graduates due to the heavier load of classes and much more intense focusing that will be required of him during his senior year.

To this day when we sit and discuss everything we went through over this five-year period, he feels that the military school had the greatest impact on him. That military school took a totally, disrespectful and apathetic kid and turned him completely around.

Here is a piece of poetry that Portlan recently wrote (I had to change a few descriptive adjectives so the content was acceptable for this book). It is one of the best examples of typical thought process in the brain of a person with ADHD. As you read this, realize that his brain is constantly working in overdrive, without a break, all day long even when he is in a class or trying to do homework.

"Ten Minutes of Me"

My body is limp, with only my right hand tense, so as to string
  together these words. Boundary-less, I never understood free
  verse until now.
I still don't.
I don't know what this is.

I walk. I stop. I write.

I just want to be held.
This overwhelming sense of desire to be needed comes over me.
I need to be validated like a parking ticket.
I need "real" love like a rabbit needs a carrot.
So, I suppose I don't really need it.
It's just my food of choice

The expanse of blue sea that I see really soothes me.
Why is it all about me?
I don't want to walk back to my room.
I want to take my shirt off and feel the breeze on my back,
    but I won't.

I'm still on campus and would be judged for doing such a thing.
Still I want to.

I am a creature of impulse.
I am a creature of habit.
It depends on what day it is.
It depends on how much my mood has swung since I have
    been asleep.

My moods are like a double-hinged door.
They can go either way, quickly.
I could be alone today and feel like the most loved person
    in the world.

I could be surrounded by those who love me tomorrow and feel meaningless.

My life is fiction.
So is yours.
I am a hypocrite.
So are you.
Now it is about both of us.

Today I messed up in school.
I don't care.
Today is not important in the scheme of my life.
Why?
Because I said so.

You and I probably don't have the same beliefs.
You also probably live more peacefully than me.

I could have kept walking to my room and never let these thoughts out of their prison.

If this letter seems coherent to you, you probably have ADHD too.

I'm a spark plug.
I need to find an engine

Did God put a warranty on my life?
If so, how long?
I wanna know when it expires so I know when I have to be more cautious.
Then again, it's possible to get cheated out of a warranty.
It's also plausible I could do "something" that is not covered by the warranty.
I wonder if recklessness could be found under the section of "somethings."

I have the will power of many men.
But I have the desire of even more men.
That makes the former useless.

I am open.
All I have the same as you is skin and bones and tendons and
muscle and nerves.
So, everything... except the electrical impulses that get sent
through our bodies.
Wow. Interesting.

I feel like crying
Because of beauty, because of pain, because of pleasure, because
of weight.

My life has weight.
I weigh 170 pounds.

[...]

Do I like who I am?
Do I?
Sometimes I do and others I don't.

How do people think of me?
Do they see my insanity and simply refuse to inform me?
Or do I seem like I have my life together?
Either way I am not sure which is the truth.
It doesn't matter anyway.

How does time work?
This is ten minutes of me.
Can I have ten minutes of you?

Portlan is constantly writing poems, short stories, or essays. An emotionally driven individual, he tends to put all of himself in his work and often writes about life experiences or dreams. Portlan has recently had a few poems published and is working on getting other works published. He is currently studying writing at Point Loma Nazarene University, in San Diego. We are extremely proud of the fine young man he has become.

Portlan

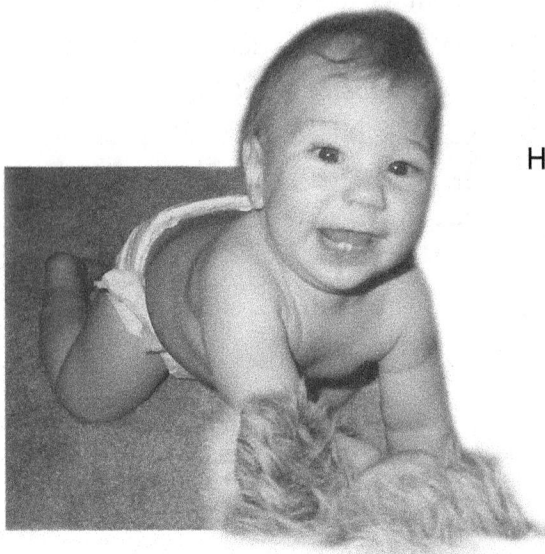

High Energy Baby
Age 6 months

Strong-Willed
Toddler
Age 18 months

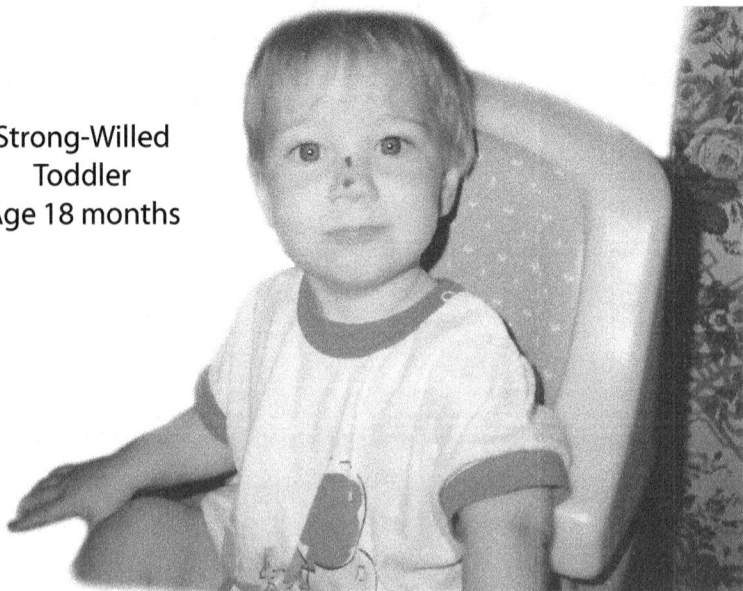

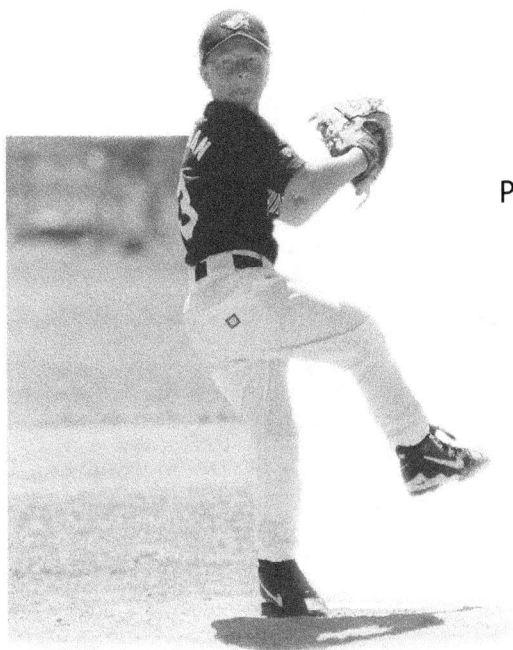

Pitching AAA
Age 10

Military School
Age 12

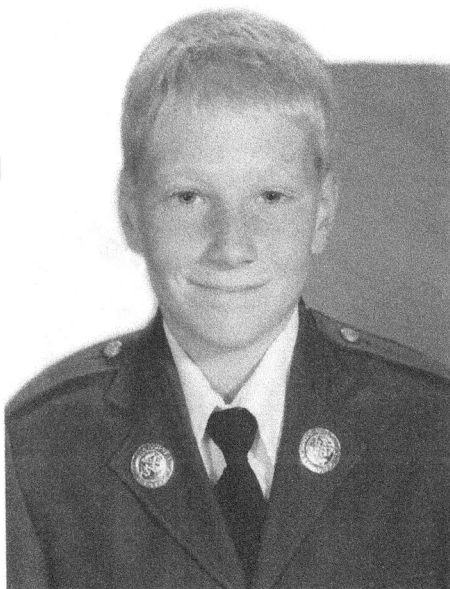

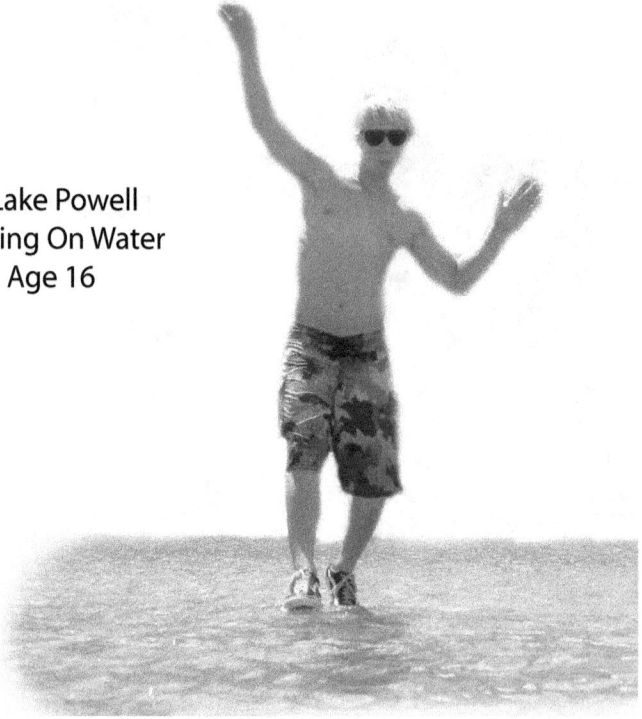

Lake Powell
Walking On Water
Age 16

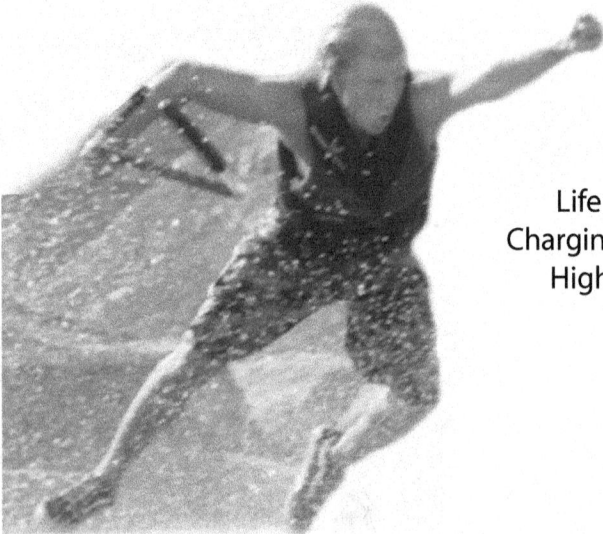

Life Is Good
Charging Ahead To
High School

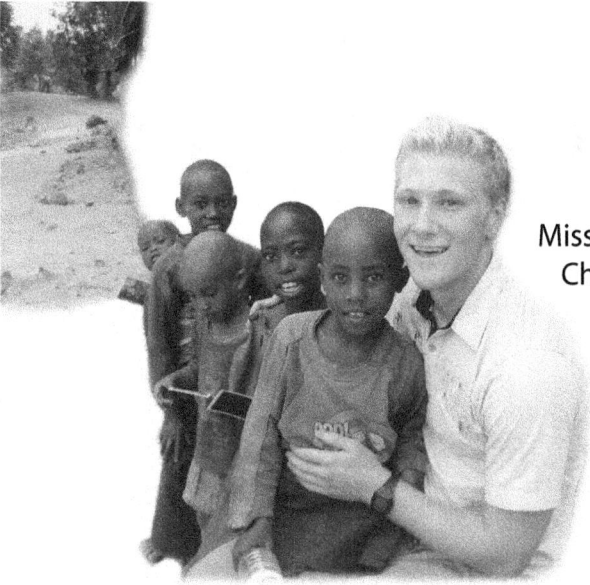

Mission Trip To Africa
Church In Rwanda
Age 18

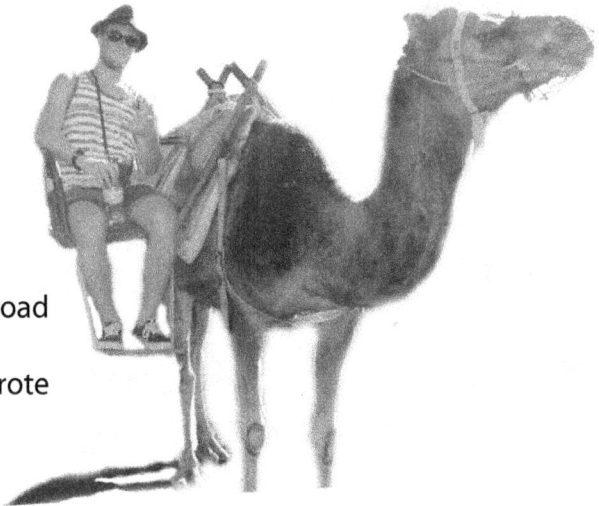

Semester Abroad
In Spain
Visiting Lanzarote
Age 20

CHAPTER 2

What Is Attention Deficit Hyperactivity Disorder (ADHD)?

T HE GENERAL UNDERSTANDING OF Attention Deficit Hyperactivity Disorder (ADHD) is the following; a disorder in which a person is unable to focus for long periods of time and has difficulty with completing tasks or projects in a timely manner. Some people have this without the hyperactivity. If they do have the hyperactivity they are similar to a motor that continues to run nonstop. They also have impulsive responses to situations in which the affected person does or says things without thinking and without being able to stop. People with ADHD are not able to consider the results of their impulsive actions and what effect they may have on themselves or the people around them.

An ADHD child continues to blurt out answers to questions in class without being chosen or sticks his or her foot out in front of someone walking by and trips them. These symptoms can first reveal themselves through children who just can't sit still and have a hard time paying attention. This describes typical behavior for most boys between the ages of four and twelve. So how do you know if your child has ADHD? Well, most of the boys who have normal symptoms of hyperactivity (ants in their pants) can get through their school work effectively and will back down to authority. A child with ADHD will have these symptoms at home, in school, and in sports. The symptoms usually show up before the kids turn seven or eight and will last for longer than a six-month period. These kids will also typically have a hard time making and keeping friends. Girls can also be diagnosed with ADHD, however boys are two to three times more likely to have it. Symptoms are the same for boys and girls.

Another disorder that many times is in conjunction with ADHD is Oppositional Defiance Disorder (ODD). People with ODD question authority and have a defiant attitude towards authoritative figures such as parents, teachers, principals, and coaches. Children with ODD are very strong-willed, difficult to discipline, and have to control every situation. They have a "my way or the highway" attitude. Often ODD is more of a symptom associated with ADHD than its own disorder. You rarely see a kid who has ODD and doesn't have ADHD.

Some statistics show that ADHD is very hereditary and most children with ADHD have at least one parent, if not both, who also suffers from it. Sometimes it can come from an uncle or an aunt who has it. Most adults who weren't diagnosed as a child don't realize they have it until their own child is diagnosed. Just as often though, the ADHD can't be traced to any family members and is just that child's "programming." A child's prenatal and or social situations can be factors that contribute to ADHD such as being adopted. Children who have been adopted are commonly considered or diagnosed with ADHD and have difficulty when they cannot relate or identify with either of their adoptive parents. Very often ADHD will be missed when a child is diagnosed with a learning disorder.

**Here is a guide to diagnosing your own child's inattention.
Does your child often:**

☐ Not pay close attention to details or make careless mistakes during school or other activities?

☐ Not listen when being spoken to directly by an adult?

☐ Have difficulty completing tasks he or she is given, such as chores, homework, getting dressed, brushing teeth, etc?

☐ Not have the ability to get organized?

☐ Lose things such as toys, homework, books, pencils, etc?

☐ Become easily distracted?

☐ Forget things?

**Here is a guide for diagnosing Hyperactivity.
Does your child often:**

☐ Have a hard time taking turns?

☐ Act as if driven by a motor unable to stop?

☐ Talk incessantly and very fast?

☐ Blurt out answers and make comments?

☐ Interrupt people while they are speaking?

☐ Constantly get up and down from his or her seat at the dinner table or in class?

☐ Have to be moving or fidgeting?

☐ Run or climb things in inappropriate situations?

☐ Show no fear in potentially dangerous situations?

If you are answering yes to most of these questions then I recommend you speak to your pediatrician or better yet a true specialist in behavior and learning problems about doing further testing on your child (see the sidebar on Testing and Results). Again, these symptoms can be applied to both boys and girls. Do not wait for a teacher to bring this to your attention, because some children don't have all the obvious symptoms. The earlier a child is diagnosed with ADHD and treated with the proper combination of behavior management (a form of discipline that is set up through a contract between the child and the parent stating the consequences of inappropriate behavior), medication, and counseling, the higher the rate of success. Parents and doctors can still get through to an eight- to twelve-year-old child versus trying to treat a fifteen- to nineteen-year-old who may already be experimenting with illegal drugs and can often become very combative during treatment. The big issue is these symptoms or problems above get in the way of a person's performance, self-esteem, and relationships.

Don't let all the myths about ADHD medication sway your decision to treat your child. Most of the medications used have been around for a very long time and have been improved. There are also many newer brands to choose, so if your child doesn't respond well to one there are many others to try. All people respond to medication differently.

Most of the kids and adults today who smoke have some form of ADHD. The nicotine in cigarettes and chewing tobacco has been found to have a similar effect that the ADHD medication methylphenidate (brand names Ritalin and Concerta) has and helps people with ADHD to calm down and focus better. There are many studies under way that are looking at the effects of nicotine on attention and concentration. According to Dr. Alexander Potter, PhD, (postdoctoral fellow, clinical Neuroscience Research unit at the University of Vermont, Burlington, USA) his test studies have noted that kids with ADHD take up smoking and become hooked at twice the rate of other adolescents. Throughout Dr. Potter's testing, nicotine proved to be just as effective at helping attention as methylphenidate, if not more.

In another study, Dr. Potter tested the impulsivity of teens with ADHD and their inability to inhibit their behavior. The teens were given a test on a computer and they all failed the test on their own, but when given nicotine they all passed the test as if normal. According to another doctor, Dr. Newhouse, there are at least three pharmaceutical companies working on novel nicotinic agents and they are "thinking of targeting ADHD" with these investigational drugs (www.docguide.com).

The problem with nicotine is that it is so addicting, and the use of tobacco can lead to cancer and many other life-threatening diseases. Also the duration of the effect is very short and there is an unacceptably large variability in dosing, "same as drinking coffee." The other problem with teens and cigarettes is the potential for them to use other, stronger drugs. According to the book *Alcoholism, Drug Addiction, and the Road to Recovery: Life on the Edge,* by Barry Stimmel (page 156), "It is stated that researchers studying marijuana use in adolescents say that experimentation with the drug sometimes leads from occasional social use to continued regular use, and finally cocaine, heroin, or hallucinogens. Almost every such study, however, has shown that alcohol and nicotine consistently preceded that kind of progression as well."

For the past ten years I have been conducting my own study. Every time I see a person smoking who is between fifteen and twenty-five years old, I ask them if they have ever heard of ADHD or know what it is. I haven't had a single smoker yet who didn't tell me immediately, "Yes I have ADHD, and I know smoking is a terrible habit, but my mom didn't believe in medication." Cigarettes have nicotine in them, and the nicotine helps with ADHD symptoms like the medicine methylphenidate does, only methylphenidate is nonaddicting and doesn't cause cancer.

The reality of children with untreated ADHD is they can develop other problems later in life, including anxiety, depression, volatile behavior, and addictions. The symptoms of ADHD can change over time. Even with developed coping skills the condition will never go completely away.

Technology and ADHD

In the next few years they will have more tools for diagnosing ADHD. Hopefully in the near future they will diagnose ADHD with magnetic resonance imaging (MRI) of the brain. An MRI shows how different the brain of an ADHD individual is compared to someone who doesn't have it.

An electroencephalogram (EEG) is a test that measures and records electrical activity in the brain. It is very rare for ADHD patients to have abnormal EEG's. There may be a distinct brain wave pattern that ADHD patients have compared to those without ADHD. There are experimental therapies using this information to help patients retrain their brain waves. This information may lead to future ways of diagnosing and treating ADHD, but it is not yet largely accepted or in use. Perhaps more scientific studies will shed more light on this subject.

The Drake Institute in Southern California uses neurofeedback to treat attention deficit disorder and other conditions without the use of medication. I have many friends that have tried neurofeedback as opposed to medication. It seems successful for a few but is extremely expensive and there are no documented studies showing a long-term benefit. It takes a lot of patience because it is definitely not a quick fix and generally requires the parents to create a setting in which their child can adapt to and learn to cope with ADHD and any other disabilities they may have. Unfortunately, we live in a world of constant change. All children continuously change as they grow and develop, therefore creating an environment that could last for your child's entire school years or life would be next to impossible and certainly not reality.

Testing and Results

The following tests measure different mental abilities and achievements and typically need to be given by a psychologist to get the best results. The tests can be very beneficial to diagnosing your child with ADHD.

The WISC-IV test is a basic measure of mental ability. All the subtests have scales and scores with a mean of 10 and a standard deviation of 3, while IQ and factor scores are presented as standard scores with a mean of 100 and a standard deviation of 15. The subtests score the verbal comprehension, perceptual reasoning, working memory, processing speed, and full scale IQ. Some of these subtests include oral responses as well as the written.

The PRI, Perceptual Reasoning Index, is designed to measure fluid reasoning in the perceptual domain with tasks that assess nonverbal concept formation, visual perception and organization, simultaneous processing, visual-motor coordination, learning, and the ability to separate figure and ground in visual stimuli.

The Working Memory Index provides information regarding the child's ability to react to something that is asked of him or her verbally, process the information in memory, and then formulate a response.

The Processing Speed Index (PSI) is designed to measure an individual's ability to process simple or routine information without making errors.

The Full Scale IQ score is then derived from a combination of the ten subtest scores and is considered the most representative estimate of global intellectual functioning.

The WIAT-II is a measure of academic achievement. In contrast to a mental ability or intelligence test, academic achievement presumes that training within a specific area has taken place. The subtests for this particular test revolve around reading, writing, and mathematics. When you take the tests and compare the results along with the IQ and the standard deviations, you can determine if there is any large discrepancy between the child's ability and his or her achievement.

The BGT-II is a perceptual-motor drawing task that requires the child to copy twelve geometric figures and patterns. This test is used as a measure of visual-motor integration skills and as a screening tool for neuropsychological dysfunction.

The BASC-2 is a behavior checklist filled out by a parent and teacher. It measures many aspects of behavior and personality, including positive (adaptive) behaviors as well as negative (clinical) dimensions.

The CWSRS is a self-reporting scale for ADHD and is filled out by the child once he or she is old enough to understand and effectively rate his or her own actions and feelings.

The MASC is a self-reporting scale for anxiety. This can only be filled out by a child who is old enough to understand the questions being asked and can give an accurate account of what he or she is feeling.

The school district will give many of the above tests for no charge whether you go to public or private school, but they often come back with inconclusive results. Some schools aren't willing to give the tests unless your child is thought to be autistic, mentally retarded, or at least two years behind in school. As a parent, begin the process of getting the testing by writing the school a letter explaining your concerns, and they have to respond to you within certain time limits. The school psychologist can give some of the tests, and you can use this as a starting point for getting your child the help he or she needs. These tests are available for free, and the results can be useful in getting your child services or extra time for tests in the classroom.

The public schools have a program, called the 504 program, which allows students to receive special services based on their level of disability or needs for extra time on tests and modified homework. There is also another program called Individualized Education Program (IEP), which is similar to the 504 and is mandated by the Individuals with Disabilities Education Act (IDEA). Unfortunately, most of the private schools do not have their own programs like these, although more and more of them are realizing that each child in a family is different and just because one sibling may be an excellent student who can excel in an advanced program the next sibling can be quite different. In order to allow families to keep all their children in the same school many private schools are starting to implement their own modified programs to help these siblings who need the extra help. Some private schools will accept and integrate the 504 program into their school program and honor IEPs.

As a mother of three children with ADHD, I have my own anxieties over finding the right treatments for this disorder. If your child were diagnosed with diabetes would you not give them insulin? Of course you would because your child would die without the insulin! Attention deficit is a valid disorder in which there is a dysfunction of the brain and which many medications can help, so I am baffled as to why so many parents choose not to medicate. No your child will not die without these medications, but the person they have the potential to become often dies unless you develop an effective treatment plan during the formative years between childhood and adolescence. Meanwhile, your child is suffering inside every day when he or she has to go to school and feel stupid compared to his or her smart peers.

Children all want to feel smart, so when they can't keep up with their peers in class they begin to lose self-confidence. These feelings build over the years and eventually they become depressed and lonely. This is when they turn to alcohol and drugs. They will also try to find friends whom they feel smart around, and these are typically not the kids you want them hanging around. Children who suffer from the symptoms of ADHD don't have to struggle throughout the school day. They need their parents to help them find a safe and legal way to function and cope with their disorder!

Finding the Right Doctor

Finding the right doctor is probably the most difficult part of ADHD, mostly because not very many child psychologists specialize in ADHD. Most psychiatrists want to work with adults. Many of the doctors who do prescribe ADHD medications get comfortable with a few medications and aren't willing to learn about all the others out there. Many pediatricians today have been forced into learning about ADHD medications because there are so many more kids being diagnosed. The problem with your pediatrician prescribing the ADHD medications is that they typically stick with the most popular medications and are not able to be of much help if those three aren't effective for your child's needs. They will not prescribe antidepressants with these meds in order to make them more effective, nor can they help you with behavioral therapies. They are also under time limitations from the insurance companies, which gives them hardly the proper amount of time to spend with each patient.

Getting the right help is a dilemma and is partially why I made my journal into a book so people could have access to all the information I was fortunate enough to get through my doctor who specializes in ADHD. There are doctors out there like mine. You just have to really search and constantly network with people who have kids with ADHD. I have found most of my information because I have always been very open about my kids' ADHD and will talk to anyone anywhere about it. You can learn from other people by opening up. My husband and my parents used to get upset with me because ADHD was all I talked about whenever we were at a party or at the park or even at Disneyland in line for a ride. But I know I have helped hundreds of people over the years just because I am willing to share all my knowledge and experience with perfect strangers, and I have gained valuable information from them as well.

Having ADHD should not be a deep dark family secret that is embarrassing and shameful. The more you share the more you grow! ADHD is something that you should be embracing not erasing. With all the medications that my kids have taken, no one ever believes me when I tell them that they take medication. My kids are very outgoing but polite and respectful. If your child is put on a medication that makes him or her dull and out of it, then it is not the correct medication. Medication should never change your child's personality. It should just help your child to learn how to respond to situations with appropriate behavior. Search for a doctor who specializes in childhood mood disorders and ADHD. They will typically have an MD after their name along with an MPH or other possible specialties. You just want to make sure they are very knowledgeable with all the ADHD meds and other possible medications that can be combined with them so your child isn't experiencing any side effects.

CHAPTER 3

A Sweet and Sensitive
Little Brother

WHEN PORTLAN WAS TWO I became pregnant with twins, but I miscarried one and that left me still pregnant with my son Payton. It was a stressful pregnancy because I had to have ultrasounds monthly to make sure the other sac was reabsorbed properly. They called it a reabsorbing twin, which I had never heard of before. Being a twin myself I was shocked that I had become pregnant with twins.

Payton was much different from his older brother from day one. He was only 6 lbs, 15 ozs, and he started screaming the minute he came out and didn't stop for four months. Payton was a very cranky baby. Every night from 8 pm to 11 pm he would cry, and there was no consoling him. He didn't sleep through the night until he was four months old. He did sleep a lot during the day though, from 10 am to 2 pm every day.

By five months old he started calming down and becoming a much happier baby. He got his first tooth at eight months old. By eighteen months he still didn't talk much, and he spoke with baby talk, which Portlan never did. Payton called Goofy,

"Foofy," and we would laugh so hard. I never realized how cute the baby talk was. When he was into his twos he became so easy for me that I didn't even know he was home. He loved to play by himself for hours and then he would oftentimes put himself down for a nap, unlike his older brother Portlan, who always needed me to play with him because he could not entertain himself.

Payton was such a joy up until he was three, especially after what Portlan put me through. He potty trained at age three, which was normal for a boy, and he finally started talking in complete sentences, so people could understand him better. The boys got along really well, which was kind of unusual, but I think the age difference helped. Once Payton reached the age of three, he started to experience temper tantrums more than I would have liked. He was extremely sensitive to many things, and once he started crying it was difficult to calm him down. If I was speaking loudly to Portlan or reprimanding him, Payton would often start crying just from the tone in my voice. His emotional roller coaster lasted all the way into kindergarten and first grade.

Our Second Diagnosis

Once we had gotten Portlan diagnosed, medicated, and settled down I noticed that Payton was having some problems. He was the polar opposite of Portlan. He was a sweet, shy, quiet, sensitive, and very respectful child. He never stepped out of line. He had always been very sensitive, starting with the colic as a baby. Getting him dressed was quite a chore because everything bugged him. I had to remove the tags from his shirts and pants. His socks drove him nuts because the seam along the toes that holds your socks together bugged him. He even wore them inside out sometimes.

Payton was very small for his age. Even though he was five and half when he started kindergarten, the private school wanted me to hold him another year. I told them no and we ended up having to take him to Portlan's new school so he could start kindergarten. He had a rough year because he was so shy and quiet. What a difference compared to Portlan. One time the teacher called me to tell me that Payton didn't know the alphabet, and I laughed and told her that was ridiculous. He wouldn't recite the alphabet for her because he was afraid that he would say one of the letters wrong, and this was extremely frustrating for her.

He managed to get through kindergarten, and for first grade he got a young, new teacher whom he really adored. He would do anything for her, and he often sat at a table that was right next to her desk because she adored him too. So he finished first grade without too many problems. But by the middle of second grade, we were noticing that he wasn't learning to read very well, and his handwriting was illegible. He was also very emotional and crying all the time. I didn't really notice how badly Payton was doing until we had gotten Portlan settled down.

We decided to get him help at the time we were with the second psychiatrist from my HMO. I happened to mention to him that Payton was very emotional and seemed to fall apart over the slightest thing. I also mentioned the hypersensitivity to everything that touched him. He told me that typically if one child has ADHD so will the sibling. I didn't see any of the same symptoms in Payton that I had seen with Portlan. But I figured it was worth a try since I didn't want him to go through all the same social issues that Portlan went through.

We tried 5 mg of Ritalin (methylphenidate) with Payton once a day. Almost immediately his mood evened out and he wasn't so sensitive about everything. Over the next few months he suddenly caught on to reading, and his printing went from the worst in the class to one of the best. We were really excited to see him become so successful in school and much happier. He finished out his second grade year with much more confidence than we had ever seen in him before.

He continued to do very well in third grade, having many good friends and enjoying school. The teachers adored his very respectful attitude, and his perfect conduct was such a joy to us. He really was a sweet child, and everyone who came into contact with him loved him. When we started seeing the new specialist, Dr. B, he recommended that we switch Payton from Ritalin to Concerta (methylphenidate) since it was a time-release medication that lasted all day. Avoiding medication with ups and downs is extremely important.

A Quick Break from Medicine

When Portlan went off to military school, Payton was starting fourth grade and was doing really well. We had decided to take him off his medication for the summer, since he really just needed it for focusing in class. We also decided to have him do the same testing that Portlan had done since we didn't have any documented testing on him. Along with the ADHD tests, I also had Payton tested for allergies since I had read somewhere that some kids can have severe allergies that can hinder their ability to focus. He tested negative to all foods and outdoor pollens, dust, grass, and mold.

Payton started fourth grade with no medication, and after about two weeks of school, he was starting to have some real issues in class. He couldn't keep up with the teacher in class or focus on any reading. After school he and I would sit and do homework for about three hours a night. It took so long because he would mostly cry and whine about how hard it was and that he couldn't write for that long.

Then I got a call from his teacher who was very concerned and bewildered because she knew how well he had done in third grade. I explained to her that he had been on medication for the last two years and we were just making sure he really needed it. I told her that he was going through some testing and that kids shouldn't be medicated during any testing so you get a true read on their skills. I let her know that as soon as the testing was over he would probably go back on his Concerta.

Once we got all the test results back and had a confirmation that Payton had ADHD without the hyperactivity he went back on the Concerta. He probably was about four weeks into the school year, and he started his medication on a Monday. Until this point I had spent four solid weeks every day after school from 3:30 to 6:30 helping him get through his homework.

On that first Monday he was back on his meds, he took his pill and went to school. I had expected that he would still need some help with his homework because it was fourth grade, which is much harder than third. When he came home that day I asked him how his day went and he told me it was great and he was very excited. He said, "Mommy when the teacher called on me in class today I knew exactly where we were, and I was able to read and answer the question she asked." I was so excited for him! Then I asked him when he wanted to get started on his homework. He looked at me, and I will never forget this day as long as I live, he said, "I don't have any home-work, I did it all during Later Gators." Later Gators was an after-school program for the kids who got out thirty minutes before the older kids. They all would go in and do homework or talk until it was time to go to pick-up with their siblings or carpool. I couldn't believe what I heard! I HAVE NEVER DONE HOMEWORK AGAIN WITH THIS CHILD.

Two days later, his teacher called me and wanted to know what we did because the change in him was so significant she couldn't believe it. When I told her that he just started back on his Concerta she couldn't believe that it could be that quick and simple.

One day driving home in the car Payton told me that there was one or two other kids in his class who had the same problems that he had without medication. He said, "Mommy why won't those kids' moms help them, because they really need help?" I explained to him that there are a lot of people who don't agree with giving their kids medication like I do. I told him that some day he may ask me why I gave him medication, but I also told him that I am doing what I feel is the right thing to do for my children. He continued to ask me why a parent wouldn't let their child take one pill if that could help them to do well in school and let the teacher and others kids see how smart they really are?

Public School and Beyond

Payton saw his brother excel in public school, and he felt that he could do much better academically as well. He asked us if he could leave the private school after sixth grade, since he also wanted to attend the public high school. My husband and I discussed Payton's request and felt that he was choosing to switch schools for the right reasons, and we were also very happy with Portlan's experience. So that next fall Payton entered the same public junior high for seventh grade that Portlan did for his second year of eighth grade. Payton was able to get straight A's there for the first time. His academic success continued on through his eighth grade year as well.

The doctor switched Payton to a newer drug called Strattera (atomoxetine HCL), which works differently from a controlled stimulant such as Adderall, Concerta, or Ritalin. Fortunately, he did well on the Strattera from about sixth grade up until his freshman year of high school.

Payton entered the same public high school as Portlan, who was then a junior. During his freshman year he wanted to try and graduate from his medication like Portlan did. He had basically straight A's, so we thought we'd give it a try because even if he dropped down a little bit that would be fine.

Unfortunately, within a month all his A's were dropping to C's, and he was feeling overwhelmed and totally unable to focus while doing his homework. He decided it was best to go back on his meds and his grades came right back up. Thank the good Lord this kid just feels fortunate that there is medication to help him stay on track with his studies.

In terms of sports, he tried wrestling like his brother, but he told us that he was not angry enough to wrestle. We had a good laugh at that because he truly is our meek and mild child. He also tried pole vaulting but has found his true love to be surfing. He is extremely good, and as a sophomore he took his brother's spot on the varsity surf team.

Because Payton was easier to medicate than Portlan and seemed to stay on the same medication and dose for so long, I had been having our pediatrician prescribe his meds for about four years to save some money, since Dr. B was not covered by our insurance. We figured out that we were spending almost $15,000 in one year when all three of the kids and my husband were seeing the very expensive doctor. We were fortunate that our pediatrician knew this doctor and felt comfortable with his diagnosis and prescribed medications. Although Dr. B is extremely expensive, we are so grateful that we have been able to afford to see him since his expertise with the ADHD meds is priceless and his office is so kid friendly compared to any of the other "pysch" doctors we saw.

During Payton's sophomore year he started to have some problems with depression. I let it go for about six months because my pediatrician said that what he was feeling was just hormones and was normal for teens his age. But after six months of Payton's depression I felt that it might be more than hormones. He had grown a lot between his freshman and sophomore year, so I figured his meds possibly needed some adjustment. We went back to Dr. B, who was also concerned, since Payton was complaining that nothing excited him anymore. He felt like he was just going through the motions. He was starting to have issues with all of his friends as well. Since these symptoms had lasted longer than six months, the doctor prescribed the antidepressant Celexa (citalopram HCl) to see if his mood improved. Dr. B also moved Payton from Strattera to the Daytrana patch (methylphenidate), since he seemed to be having a much harder time focusing in class and while doing homework.

Within a week Payton was feeling much better and was more talkative than I had ever seen him before. He was excited to surf and play his guitar again, and he was able to concentrate much better in school and with his homework. He went on to accomplish his goal of being in a band at church and started writing his own music and lyrics. He also took up photography, for which he seems to have a natural gift and now takes amazing photos everywhere he goes. He went on his first out-of-country mission trip to the Dominican Republic with the church youth group the summer before his senior year of high school. He too has a compassionate heart for the children and people of impoverished nations in the world.

Payton managed to stay on track with school and was accepted to the same private Christian college as his brother, majoring in graphic design. Payton came to me two months before he graduated from high school, and, I will never forget this, he said, "Mom, I am so thankful that you were willing to give me medication, because I probably wouldn't have graduated from high school, and I definitely wouldn't be going to this good of a college without it, so thank you!" Moments like that are priceless for me because I am just so grateful that I made the right choice for my child. As parents we have to sometimes make very difficult decisions for our children and it is hard to know if we are doing what is best for them. I don't like to think of the medication as a crutch that my children need to be successful, but it is certainly a tool that they have been able to use so they can tap into their amazing talents and gifts. Payton to this day has a hard time when he sees kids who suffer with ADHD and are not getting the help they need from their parents.

Payton just completed his first year of college and earned a 3.0 GPA while making the surf team and working twenty hours a week. He is going to go abroad for the first semester of his sophomore year, and we couldn't be prouder of him!

Payton

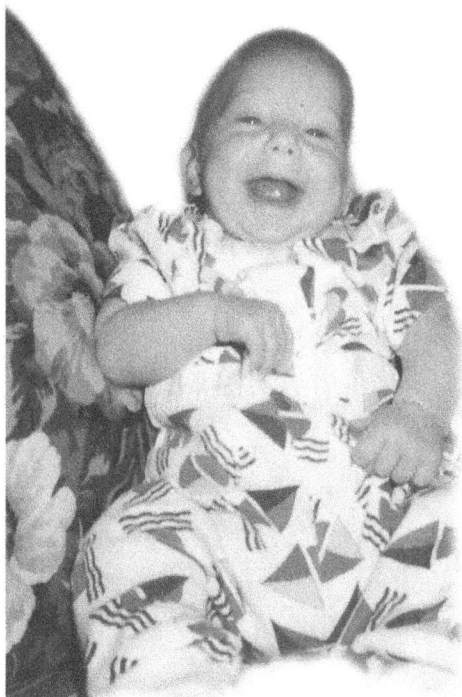

Happy At Last
Age 5 months

Sweet and Sensitive
Age 18 months

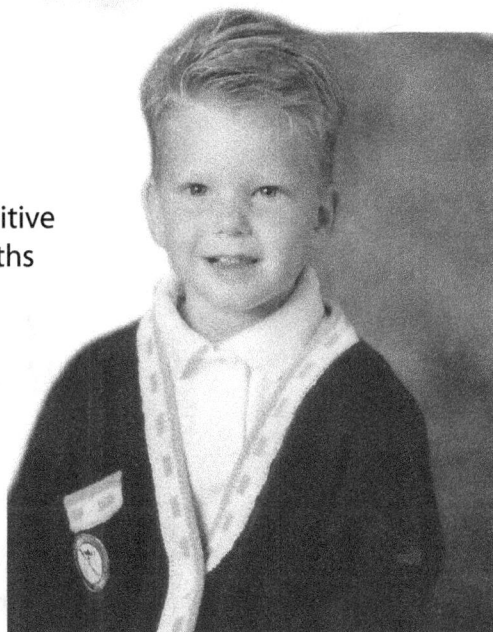

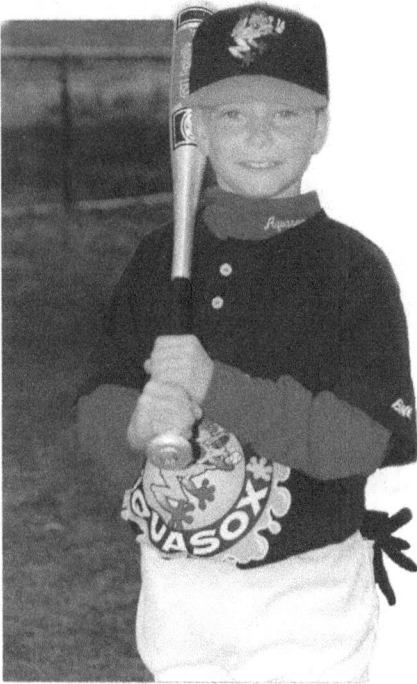

Hypersensitive
Playing AA
Age 8

Life Is Good
At Shaver Lake
Age 10

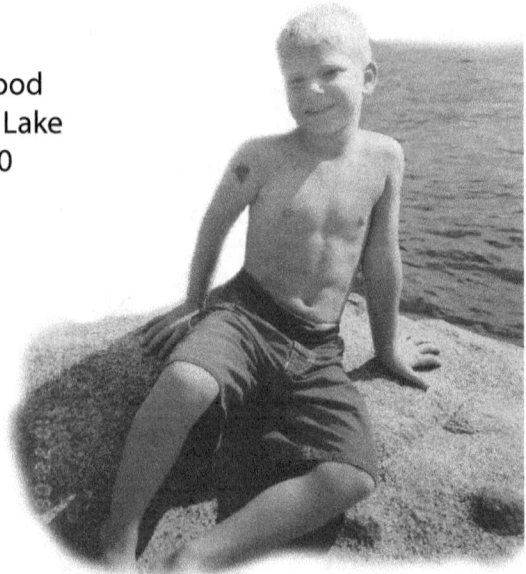

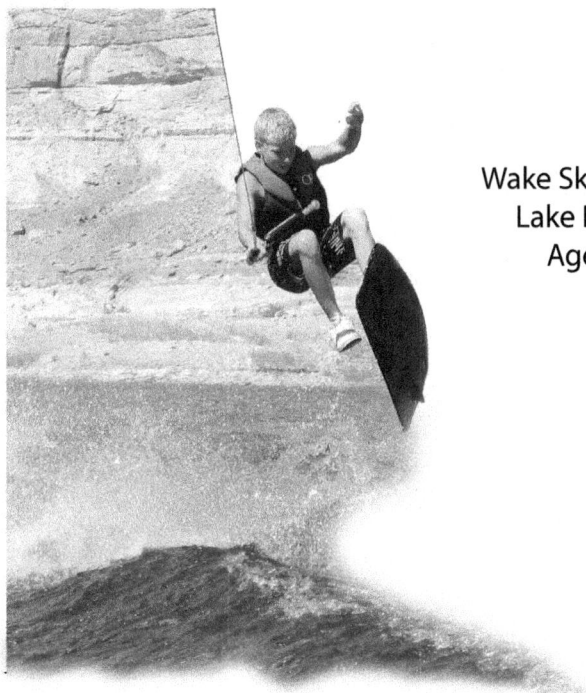

Wake Skating On
Lake Powell
Age 13

At Bass Lake
Cruising In High School
Age 17

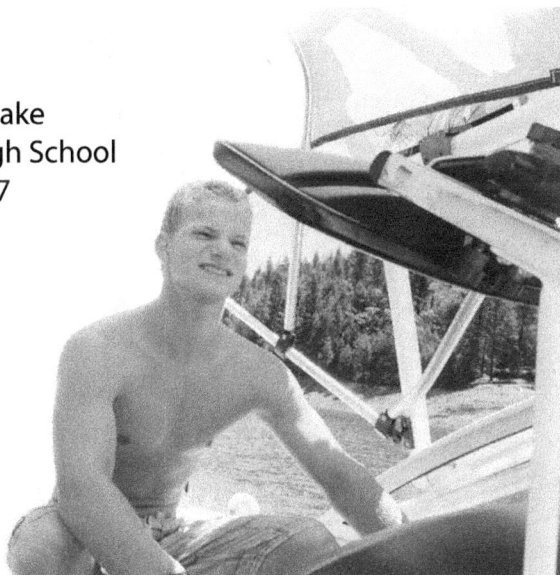

CHAPTER 4

A Joyful, Bouncing Baby Sister

PORTLAN WAS IN FIRST grade and Payton in preschool when Phoebe was born. The boys were quite a handful and I knew three boys would have put me over the top. God felt we needed a little girl to complete this family, so along came Phoebe.

Once our beautiful, bouncing baby girl came along at 7 lbs., all of our lives were changed forever. The boys immediately adored her, especially Portlan, who really wanted a sister. Payton would have liked a baby brother so he could pick on him like his brother was starting to do to him. Phoebe was a very easygoing baby and was able to just go with the flow since she spent most of her time in the car. All of my children at birth were deemed perfect and normal according to all the tests that could be run on them.

The most difficult part of having a baby with two older siblings in school was all the germs that came home with them. Phoebe managed to have chronic ear infections from about four months old. By the time she was eight months she had been on at least five different antibiotics that worked while she was taking them, but the minute she stopped the ear infections came back. At eight months we had tubes put in her tiny little ears, and they were a miracle cure. She never had another ear infection and the tubes had to be removed from her ears when she was two because they never fell out.

Phoebe followed the same growth pattern as Portlan, got her teeth early, and spoke early too. But she was also like Payton in that she too had some baby talk. She was a good sleeper and took great naps. She was my earliest walker. She took her first steps on her one-year birthday and never looked back. She was a very mild but active toddler and tried to show her power during potty training. But by that point I had some experience, and she was a girl so she was supposed to master this earlier than the boys. She tried to put up a power struggle with this, but I just stopped buying diapers and told her she could wet her new princess underwear. That pretty much took care of that power struggle.

Our Third Diagnosis

Phoebe made it through kindergarten with some of the similar struggles with reading and writing as Payton, but she was much more social and outgoing. The teacher almost considered holding her back but then changed her mind. Dr. B all along kept telling me that boys are much more likely to get ADHD than girls, so she probably wouldn't have it. She didn't have any of the same characteristics of Portlan, and she was definitely more outgoing than Payton, so it had been hard to tell if she would have it.

Within the first few weeks of first grade I was beginning to worry about her. She was having trouble learning to read, and her writing was very illegible like Payton's. She was starting to show signs of sensitivity with tags in her clothing and especially her socks. So I made an appointment for her with Dr. B and brought her in so he could examine her.

He decided that since her brothers both had ADHD (and by now we had diagnosed my husband with ADHD as well), she was probably going to need some help. He started her on a very low dose of Adderall (1/2 of a .5 mg pill), which she took in the morning before she went to school. I spoke to her teacher about it and told her that I would need her input to see if she noticed a considerable change in her.

Well, just like Payton, she immediately started writing much better, and she really improved with her reading. When we met for her parent-teacher conference that October, her teacher could not believe the difference in her. She told me that she didn't think that Phoebe would get as far as she was at that conference time by the end of the year. The teacher was amazed by the progress she made in two months with such a small dose of Adderall. Of course then she wanted to know why all the hyperactive boys in the class weren't being put on something. I explained to her that if Phoebe were my first child no doctor would have put her on medication. Only because she was a third child and she had siblings and a parent with ADHD was she able to be diagnosed and medicated.

Now, some people might find this disturbing that I was okay with medicating children so young. You might notice through this book that Payton never had any of the social issues that Portlan had at this age and Phoebe never has had them either. Portlan didn't have learning issues; his most severe symptoms were emotional. But because I didn't get him on medication until he was ten, he had already realized that he was different and had a very hard time fitting in and making friends. Payton and Phoebe never had any social issues with their peers, and they were young enough that they just took their pill with their vitamins and considered it another vitamin. They basically were too young to be labeled by themselves, peers, or teachers.

Phoebe finished first grade with flying colors and loved school. She was very social and loved all her friends and teachers. She joined a cheer gym in the second grade and was a flyer. She had a hard time learning the dance routines to her cheers, but thanks to her medication it gave her the focusing ability to learn the steps.

When Payton switched over to Strattera, Dr. B also switched Phoebe to this same medication. She was in second grade when we changed it and she stayed on it until fourth grade.

Phoebe was never tested like the boys were, but since she had so many symptoms that were associated with ADHD she was treated for ADHD. I could tell immediately when her medication wore off because she would become a bouncing ball and talk so fast that it sounded like a record on fast forward.

In fourth grade, because the academics jumped quite a bit from third, Phoebe started having a difficult time staying on track and doing her homework. Once again Dr. B switched her to Concerta, since it had been very effective with her brothers. This is where Phoebe was a lot like Portlan: when she started the Concerta she became quite agitated and more emotional. So the doctor added a second medication called Zoloft (sertraline), which helped to calm her temper and keep her more even on the Concerta. By the fourth grade all three kids had been prescribed Concerta, which seemed to be the most effective drug for them during those years.

Phoebe Enters Public School

Phoebe sailed through the rest of fourth and fifth grade. When she entered sixth grade she started to feel the need to try public school like her brothers. Fortunately, our neighborhood elementary school had been expanded to a middle school. This meant much smaller class sizes because most of the kids who had been there since kindergarten wanted to go to the bigger impacted middle school. For seventh grade, we let Phoebe leave the private school and attend this new public middle school. Her best friend Mary was there too, and Phoebe was very excited that they could finally go to school together. There were only 75 kids in her entire class and about 120 in the class below hers. It still felt like a private school without uniforms, and she was happy about that. Phoebe, like her brothers, was amazingly successful in the public school. She continued on her Concerta and Zoloft up until she started her freshman year of high school.

The summer before high school, her hormones really kicked in, and that combined with a terrible menstrual cycle meant we had to change all her meds. She developed some serious anxiety and fear, which she gets from my side of the family. She had tried just about all of the forms of methylphenidate, and none of them worked without her being irritated constantly. She was experiencing such severe anxiety that she really didn't want to leave the house or be home alone.

Dr. B finally prescribed a drug called Nuvigil (armodafinil), which is an alerting medication taken by nurses or other people who have to work twenty-four-hour shifts or split shifts. It is not a narcotic, and it has worked extremely well for her. She also stopped taking Zoloft and switched to Lexapro (escitalopram oxalate), and the doctor added Klonopin (clonazepam), which really helped her with her anxiety. She also takes Ambien (zolpidem) to get to sleep every night since her overactive mind will not let her fall asleep. This is not the Ambien CR, which is a much stronger drug that keeps you asleep and has much stronger side effects. Phoebe just takes the regular Ambien, which helps you to fall asleep and then wears off. The mixing of meds is called "titrating" which is a term used in chemistry. The use of the anti-depressants along with the stimulants helps to off set the uncomfortable side effects from the stimulants. Often it does take a few different changes in the meds to get the dosage just right. Many times depending on the phase of life and the factors that may be driving certain emotions as you saw with Phoebe can cause a complete change in meds. This is why it is so critical to be with a doctor who specializes in childhood disorders and is very familiar with all the medications available and not just two or three.

A Cheerleader's Nightmare

Phoebe made the cheerleading team her freshman year. Unfortunately, Phoebe found out that she had a fractured foot right after cheer tryouts. The doctor put her in a boot, and she was supposed to stay off it for six to eight weeks. She had made the JV cheer squad, which was both exciting and terrifying for her. She was one of the main flyers, and the flyers take on a lot of the pressure during the stunt routines. Cheer camp was coming up and she was expected to be there even with her foot in a boot. When she got to camp her coach saw that she was in a boot and asked her if she could just take it off while flying so that her stunt group could practice the new routines. She was so nervous that she was going to lose her spot on the team that she agreed to help out during the routines and take her boot off. The first day at camp they were all stretching and since she hadn't been able to practice for about four weeks already she was pretty tight. While stretching her hamstrings someone walked up behind her and pushed her leg out farther than was comfortable tearing her hamstring at the insertion. Even with both of these injuries she continued to practice with her team and didn't let anyone know how much pain she was in.

The stress from these injuries and the pressure to perform with injuries proved to be more than she could handle and definitely contributed to her high anxiety starting her freshman year of high school. Unfortunately, her injuries were so stressful on her body that she was not even physically able to try out for cheer the following May (tryouts for sophomore year).

Phoebe went into her sophomore year with no sport, and even though she was relieved to not have so much pressure on her she felt lost without cheer. She had been on a club cheer team since second grade and this was the first time in eight years that she was not on any team. She was like a fish out of water and she definitely experienced some depression. As usual she threw herself into her studies and took AP World History along with joining about five different clubs on campus. By the second semester of her sophomore year she and some of her friends decided to join the swim team. Her doctors told her that this would be great for her weakened back, and it is the only noncontact and nonimpact sport available. We were so proud of her to try something that she had never done before.

At this time the ADHD doctor wanted to change her medications and take her off of the Nuvigil and add the drug Wellbutrin (bupropion). This drug works well on anxiety and ADHD symptoms. She was able to back off the Klonopin so that she now just takes 300 mg of Wellbutrin and 10mg of Lexapro. She really liked the swim team and plans to be on the team again next spring.

Phoebe finished her sophomore year of high school with much success and is looking forward to having the freedom that comes with driving. She is going on her first out-of-country mission trip to Costa Rica with her church youth group. Just like her brothers, she has a compassionate heart and loves to serve less-fortunate children and people in less-fortunate areas of the world. She traveled to New Mexico to help paint houses and minister to people living on an Indian Reservation. She loves working with special needs children and wants to be a special education teacher. She truly has a gift with these children and they love her. Like Portlan, Phoebe's church youth group friends made a huge difference in her life. She is so grateful to have her strong faith and friends from church. She has many friends, loves school, is involved with many clubs and is happy. As parents we should strive for our children, to be able to adapt to their environment so they feel good about themselves and are accepted by their peers.

Individualized Education Program (IEP) and 504 Program

I had Phoebe use the IEP program at her high school due to severe test anxiety. This program is for kids who have ADHD or other learning disabilities and need their curriculum modified. There is also a program called the 504 for kids who have more severe learning disabilities and need a modified homework and test plan along with un-timed testing. Phoebe did not want to be put into this program even though she has test anxiety and really struggles with math and science. For more information regarding the rights of your child and their disabilities there is a great deal of information at this Website: www2.ed.gov/about/offices/list/ocr/504faq.html.

When I approached the school counselor and psychologist about the 504 program, they were surprised because Phoebe's grades were pretty good even with taking some advanced classes. They suggested that she use the IEP program since she doesn't have any learning disabilities and just has focusing issues and test anxiety. While going through the college application process with her brothers I learned that having ADHD cannot help or hurt you when applying to a college. We decided that having Phoebe in the IEP would help her succeed in the classes that she really struggles in and especially for getting extra time when taking tests.

My sons were not part of the 504 or IEP program, and Payton really could have used it. He definitely needed extra time and short breaks while taking the SAT and ACT, but because he had never been in the 504 or IEP program they wouldn't allow him to have any accommodations during his SAT or ACT tests. Even though I had all the proper documentation to prove that he had ADHD, without the school having any documentation of him being in one of these programs the college boards would not allow him the modifications that he really needed to perform his best on these tests.

Now that Phoebe is in the IEP Program and doing well with it we had to have her tested for ADHD through a psychologist. The college boards require that a student have testing done within three years of the student's graduation date from high school. Therefore, even if we had tested Phoebe in fourth grade, we would have had to do it again. She is preparing to take the AP World History test at the end of her sophomore year and we are applying to get her extra time and breaks to help alleviate her test anxiety. We had to have a psycho-educational assessment written up with all the results from her tests, which included; the Wechsler Intelligence Scale for Children Fourth Edition (WISC-IV), Wechsler Individual Achievement Test Second Edition (WIAT-II), Bender Gestalt Test Second Edition (BGT-II). Behavior Checklists: Behavioral Assessment System for Children, Second Edition (BASC-2), Conners-Wells' Self-Report Scale (CWSRS); Multidimensional Anxiety Scale for

Children (MASC). Please refer to the Testing and Results sidebar in Chapter 2, which explains what all these test results can tell you about your child. These tests are expensive when given by a licensed psychologist, and with the written assessment, they can run anywhere from $1,000 to $1,500.

The good news is if the College Board accepts this assessment and approves your child's request for the special accommodations he or she needs for any college-type test (e.g., AP Exams, SAT, or ACT) then you are done! The College Board will allow these special accommodations for any testing that is required by any college, and this accommodation will follow your child to the college he or she chooses to attend. He or she will be given these same accommodations for college classes and finals.

Phoebe

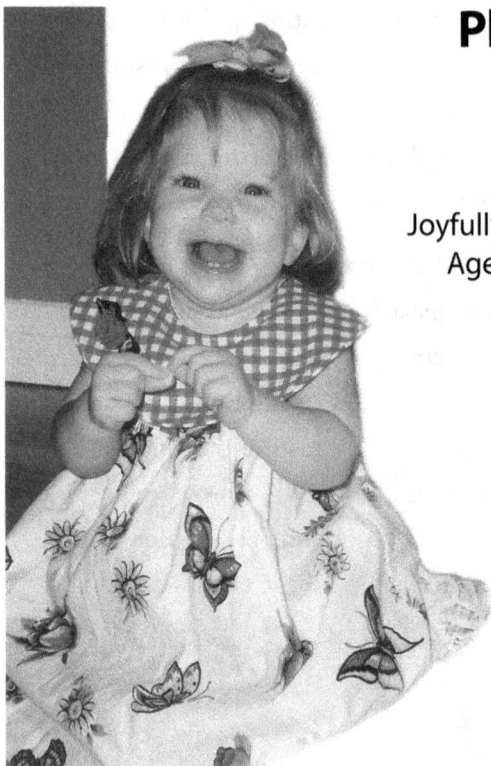

Joyfully On The Move
Age 12 months

Fearless Love For
All Creatures
Age 5

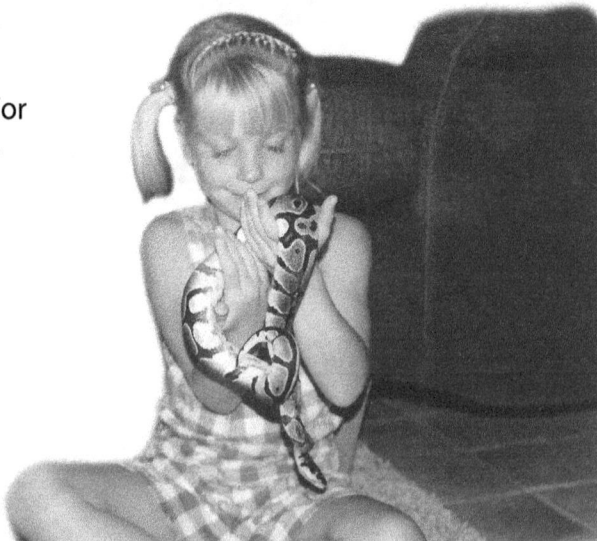

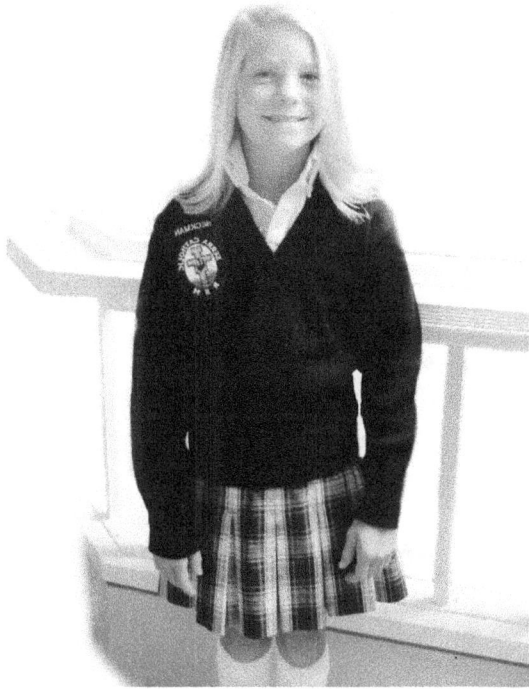

**6th Grade
Age 11**

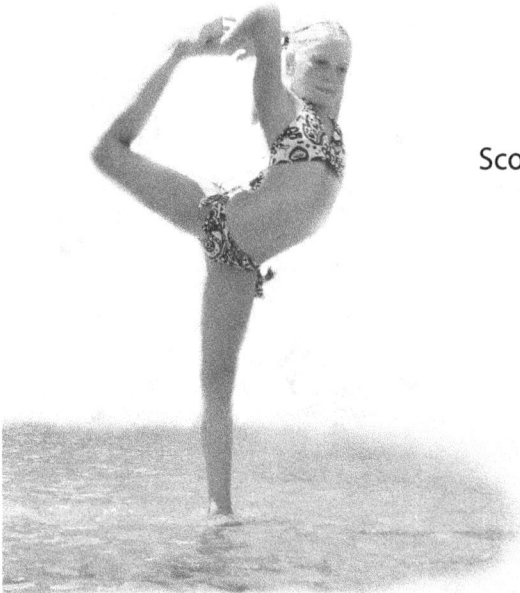

**Scorpion On Water
Lake Powell
Age 10**

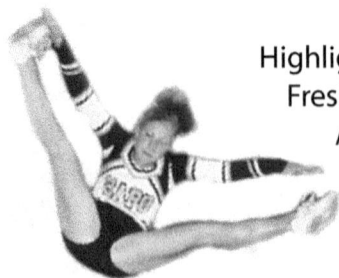

Highlight Of Cheer
Freshman Year
Age 14

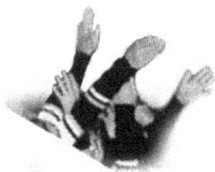

Last Winter Formal
Together,
Before Dates Arrive
Ages 14 & 18

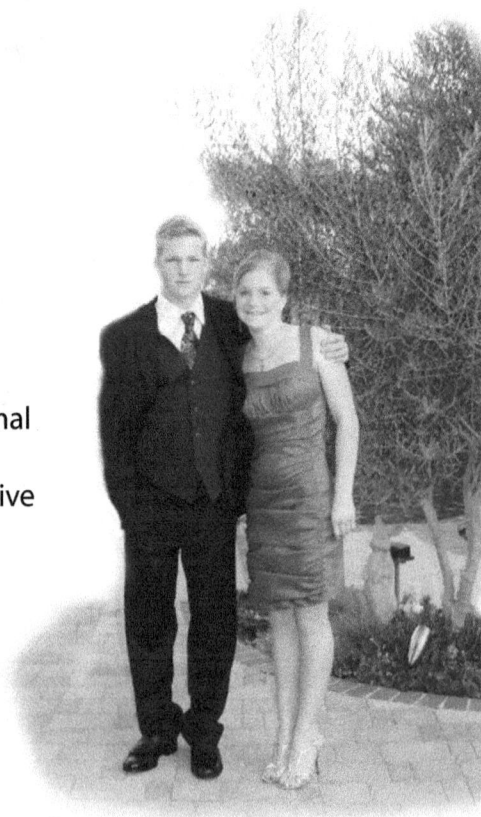

CHAPTER 5

The Power of Prayer

I RECOMMEND PRAYING OUT LOUD with your children. As a Christian mother, I can honestly say that I couldn't have gotten through what I did without the power of prayer. I firmly believe that no matter what religion you do or do not practice, just taking the time to pray can reduce the stress you take on as a parent. As our pastor Rick Warren would say, "You can choose to panic or pray, worry or worship. So if you're praying, you can't be worrying!" My main prayer for the first fifteen years of marriage was for patience, which I can honestly say saved my marriage, kids, and sanity. I was in a mothers' church group, and my children could actually tell the difference between when I was attending these meetings and when I wasn't. At one of the meetings a woman came and spoke to us about praying out loud with our children. She was much older than us, and at first I was shocked by her recommendation.

I had never prayed out loud with anyone, and I wasn't sure if my children would even like doing that. But I thought it could be a good way to get them to bed on time. Well the first night that I was going to pray I told my children after dinner what we were going to do. At this time I believe they were ten, eight, and four. I explained to them that I was going to try something new during Lent; I told them I would like to come in and pray out loud with each of them before they went to sleep. I received an overwhelming response from them. That night they all got ready for bed as fast as they could and then they stood at their doors and said, "Okay Mommy we are ready."

I started with Portlan since he was ready first, and I was so nervous. I knelt down next to his bed and held his hands while he lay in bed. I just started talking to God and asking that he help Portlan with his ADHD and to help give him the strength to be truthful. I think I prayed for about fifteen minutes. I surprised myself. When I finished I asked Portlan if he wanted to pray about anything, and he prayed for understanding and God's help with his self control.

I ended up spending about twenty to thirty minutes in each of my children's rooms that first night, and I continued to do this for the forty days of Lent that year. My husband joined in too. He would pray with a different child each night so that it didn't take me so long to get everyone to bed. My children really enjoyed praying with us, and I think it really helped them to know what things we as parents were struggling with and how much we really cared for them, and trusted God to protect them from harm. This was a really great experience for my children and one they will never forget.

CHAPTER 6

Daddy and Hubby Makes Four

I MENTIONED EARLIER THAT WE diagnosed my husband with ADHD as well, but that one took a while. He really fought the idea that he might have something that was so hereditary that he could have given it to all three children. So we had to play the "Blame Game" for a while. He started asking me all kinds of questions about how I did in school and my twin sister too. He also wanted to know more about my parents and their siblings. I understood that it was hard for him to be diagnosed with something he had had his whole life and did not realize it, and worse that was so hereditary. He came from a family of five kids and he was the baby. Out of the five kids, three have some form of ADHD.

Fortunately for him, he was more like my daughter growing up. He was outgoing, social, and hyper, but he wasn't too over the top. He had a hard time learning to read, but he developed some really good coping skills along the way. He told me one time that he was actually more shy and introverted however, he wanted to be more outgoing so he forced himself to be more social.

By the time he got to high school he was having focusing issues and began chewing tobacco. He used tobacco all through high school and college to get through his tough focusing times. He has always had a problem with being on time since our very first date in 1982. He is always running about an hour late and he can't leave work when he says he is to save his own life. Or maybe he is saving his life by leaving so late every day, I don't know.

Now, when I first met him I just thought he had too much on his plate and that was why he was always late. As the years went by I just thought it was a bad habit and it kind of became a joke with my family. On our wedding day his schedule had him showing up an hour earlier than he needed to be there to ensure he didn't miss our wedding. Once married, he seemed to start a lot of projects, but he never quite finished them. I still thought all these characteristics were just things he needed to work on and some day he would change.

Jump forward through fifteen years of marriage and three kids who all have been diagnosed with ADHD. At that time, someone recommended to us a book called *Driven to Distraction*. I thought that my husband should read it, but he has a hard time reading books in his free time! So on one of our lake trips I decided I was going to read the book aloud to him while he was driving and see what he thought. I managed to read the whole book to him by the time we got home. The book is about an adult who has ADHD and the person is talking about all the things that are difficult to accomplish at work and at home. Of course, as I was reading this book to my husband I couldn't believe how much this person was like him, but I never said anything. About a month later he came to me and said, "I have been thinking a lot about that book you read me, and I could really relate to the person in that book. I think I do have ADHD."

He decided to start seeing the kids' doctor, Dr. B, to see if he could figure out a way to handle work and life in general better. He was beginning to develop a short temper that would come out in a rage with the kids and me, but it came out of frustration more than anything else. He was still late all the time, and his office at work was very disorganized with piles everywhere. I had managed to get all the kids under control and happy with their lives, and I could see he was in need of some help too.

He tried some different medications, but he had a hard time finding something that agreed with him. He had some anxiety going on, and Ritalin can make that worse. He started using Daytrana patches, which can have fewer side effects since the transdermal patches are much easier to handle than the pills. It lasts all day long and it is also a form of the ingredient in Ritalin (methylphenidate). He also tried a few antidepressants before settling with Celexa, which keeps his mood more even and helps him to sleep. He could not have functioned properly in the job he had at that time without medication. He is no longer with that company and has since been able to get back into a regular exercise program and a better diet.

He was able to stop the Daytrana and is now trying to get his own company off the ground. He has wanted to do this for the last fifteen years and just hasn't had the financial freedom to do it. He has had all the information to write his own book over the last twenty years, written on pieces of paper here and there, and hopefully one day he will get it written. He is also a gifted writer when it comes to poetry, the apple doesn't fall far from the tree (Portlan). The kids get all their gifted writing skills and creativity from him. My husband has the ability to come up with unlimited ideas in a very short period of time and expand on them, but he needs a partner who can do the implementation part of it.

I have explained to all my kids that if they choose a career that matches their energy level and natural gifts then they should be able to stop taking medication once they are out of school. The most difficult problem people have with ADHD is performing tasks that do not interest them or are possibly too dry and mundane to hold their attention.

My husband's perfect job is outside sales simply because he is in different offices with different people everyday and he builds relationships quickly. We are hoping and praying that his new business venture is successful and allows him to fulfill his purpose and passion in life as well. He has always been successful in business due to his uncompromising values, genuine interest in helping others and persistence. His unlimited energy and ability to adjust to any situation are just a few of the benefits of his ADHD.

Marriage and ADHD

Many marriages with spouses and children who have ADHD end in divorce. We have been married for twenty-five years and it has taken a lot of patience and compromise! We have also used marriage counseling a few times through the years when we felt we weren't communicating effectively. I have definitely had to find ways to cope with my husband's tardiness and disorganization, especially with my type A personality. On the other side, he has also had to make adjustments in living with a control freak and hyper-organized person who is always three steps ahead of him. Fortunately, we were college sweethearts and what I like to think of as true soul mates. We have been very committed to making this marriage work, and we have always put each other first and the kids second. We had a priest recommend that we put our marriage first when we were engaged, which shocked me. Now our kids are leaving home, and it will soon be just the two of us again. Thankfully, we have worked hard to keep our relationship strong and we are looking forward to the next chapter in our lives as we continue on our wonderful journey.

Communication is the key to any relationship. As long as both of you are talking, listening, and feeling compassion for the person you are communicating with, you should be able to work through the issues. My husband and I have had to work really hard at that, especially during those times when we both were in need of some compassion from each other at the same time! You owe it to your children to keep your marriage strong and healthy, but at the end of the day you really owe it to yourselves. Kids today feel way too much entitlement, and we as parents often make their lives too easy. We have to be living examples of how to pull through the tough times without giving up or throwing in the towel. My husband and I have shown our kids how hard we have to work at our marriage, but we also show them how much we love each other and our marriage.

Surviving the waves of ADHD all comes down to ENDURANCE! The beaches near our home can expect waves every single day, but it depends on which way each beach faces as to how big or small those waves are going to break. Now that my husband and I have seen all the successes of our kids and celebrated twenty-five years of marriage, we know no matter how hard the waves are breaking we can face them together and endure their force!

CHAPTER 7

My Childhood and Coping Skills

B ASED ON MY OWN upbringing, I had my own quirks and challenges in raising my family. Both of my parents are organized, so I guess I get that gene from both of them. I was raised in a home in which we were not even able to leave folded clothes sitting out in our room let alone dirty ones. My bedroom looked like it was ready to be photographed for Home Magazine 24-7, and we were not able to bring kids in and out of the house. We even had to wipe the water out of the sink if we washed our hands.

Fortunately, despite growing up in a structured home, I also got my father's more laidback personality and sense of humor, so I was not fazed by having a houseful of eight boys, Phoebe with her girlfriends, and some barking dogs in the house all at the same time. I definitely learned to embrace the commotion in our house. My kids have always loved to play outside more than any other kids on our block, which is how it was when I grew up. We didn't sit inside getting addicted to video games and watching five to six hours of TV a day. Our kids have always been happier on the move, so they were always able to use their creativity to keep busy all day long. This activity is the part of ADHD that I truly embrace and love!

I am thankful for the control component I received from my mother that made me keep searching for answers about ADHD so that I could help our kids in the areas of their lives where they struggle. I have always managed to create a very organized and clean environment in the house for my husband and kids. Because of the way my mother was as I was growing up, I realized that some things are just over the top. Still I could not leave my house every morning unless everyone's beds were made and their rooms neat and clean. Since I had the realization that clean rooms were for my benefit and not so much my children's I did not mind cleaning their rooms. This caused some arguments with my husband, who always felt that the kids should be responsible for cleaning their own rooms and should do chores each day. Remember the part of ADHD in which a person can't complete even simple tasks? Since my kids could barely get themselves dressed and their teeth brushed before going to school, doing chores was an exercise in me following them around and making sure they did them. Following whining children around while yelling at them was not really helpful for them or me. We tried making charts with stickers, and they would get all excited when we were making the charts. Yet within three days, they were over the stickers they got for doing their chores.

My theory on keeping my kids' environment clean and organized was that some day when they left for college they would be so used to their bed being made and everything in their rooms having a place that they would not be able to handle a messy room. Well it actually worked! Portlan is an absolute neat freak when he is not at home, and Payton's roommates his freshman year of college, were so messy that he had to change rooms for the second semester. Payton's side of the room looked like it belonged to a lieutenant in the army, because it was so neat and organized. They both actually washed their sheets more than twice during the semester, which is impressive for boys!

I am not saying to every mom out there that it is your responsibility to keep your child's room immaculate. I am suggesting that you choose your battles. If you and your children don't care if their room is a disaster then leave it that way. For the obsessive-compulsive mom, I would recommend you do it for them to make your life easier. Fortunately, I have always been great at multitasking, and that is probably why it was so easy for me to keep up with all my daily chores and three busy children, toddlers through teens. I was able to find time to even play on a tennis team and meet my husband for lunch.

My Own Battle with Anxiety

I have not been able to escape all I have been through without my own medication. My mother suffers from manic depression along with generalized anxiety disorder. Thankfully, I did not get the manic depression but I do suffer from generalized anxiety disorder. I was always very anxious growing up, and I had a lot of fears. I never really slept well most of my life. Back when we were trying to diagnose Portlan, I had a minor surgery and then one of my best friends was diagnosed with breast cancer. I called it the "perfect storm." I was dealing with so much fear from so many different emotions that I started having panic attacks. I never really got overly panicked because I knew exactly what was happening, since I watched my mother have panic attacks on countless occasions. I tried exercising more rigorously to work the underlying anxiety out of me, and my mother gave me some tips on distraction and meditation. Unfortunately, nothing was working well and I found myself less and less comfortable leaving the house. I got to the point where I could barely go pick the kids up from school, and then I needed to come right back home. I wasn't sleeping or eating, and by the time we went to meet with Dr. B I was drowning in fear and anxiety. He noticed that I was not doing so well on that first visit and knew that in order for our family to function properly I needed to get past all the anxiety.

Dr. B prescribed me Remeron (mirtazapine), which is an antidepressant that works well on anxiety. Within a few weeks I was feeling much better. I stayed on this medication for almost two years and felt the best I had ever felt in my life. The anxiety was completely gone. One of the negative side effects to this medication is that it slows down the metabolism, so the patient can experience extreme weight gain. I did eventually stop taking the medication due to the weight gain on my petite stature.

I share my medical history because I feel it is important for other parents to know that even mothers sometimes need medication to make it through a crisis or tough time in their life. Just because you take medication that doesn't mean you are weak or incapable. We as parents are under so much pressure today and tend to take on way too much. All this pressure leads to too much stress, which eventually breaks even the healthiest person. So make sure you take care of yourself, so that you can take care of your family!

CHAPTER 8

Some Motherly Advice

EVERY CHILD WANTS TO be a good student. Even the "bad" kids really want to be good students. But when kids see how the majority of children in a classroom setting are able to understand what is taught and get the homework done without too much hassle, they get frustrated if they feel like the only kid who can't get it done. Don't be the parent in denial who isn't helping his or her child. Denial is probably the biggest reason most kids don't get help. The second reason they don't get help is that their parents think it's a phase and the kids will grow out of it. By the time kids should be growing out of it, parents realize that the kids really do need help, then it is typically too late.

If you think something is going on with your child, it doesn't hurt to check it out. Better to be sure that your child is staying on track so that he or she isn't involved in a train wreck. And never wait for a teacher to diagnose your child. I have heard over and over from parents, "The teacher never told me he or she had ADHD." It isn't up to teachers to decide if your child has ADHD; they are not trained doctors or psychologists.

Here is a message for all dads: STOP TREATING your child like the child you WISH they were and ACCEPT them for the child they ACTUALLY ARE! Dads have the most difficulty accepting their child having a disability or disorder, especially when it requires taking medications or needing extra help with special accommodations.

To all parents, just know your children and talk to them. Even if they are boys who don't like to talk, make them talk to you. If you are honest and open with your children, they will be honest and open with you. Kids know when their parents are trying to pull one over on them. Some people tell me that they don't agree with parents being so open with their kids, yet they want to know everything that is going on with their own kid.

My parents always answered our questions and would talk about anything. This made me feel very comfortable talking to them about issues that most kids wouldn't discuss with a parent. To this day, as a grown adult I can talk to my parents about anything, and they have transferred that same relationship to their grandchildren. My kids love to be around their grandparents because they are so easy to talk to and they can discuss any subject with them. If you want your children to want to be around you, then talk to them so they will want to talk and be around you! My two boys were both so different. Portlan loved to share everything, but I had to weed out the truth in much of what he told me for about five years. Payton was very quiet and didn't like to talk, so I really had to pull it out of him. Some days I feel like *I* have ADHD, and I jokingly tell people that I feel like I have contracted ADHD from my family. I do love how active our family is and they have all helped me to do things that I thought I could not do on our many ADHD high-activity vacations we have taken all over the world! I can honestly say that I "embrace" all the ADHD in my family, and I hope that you can learn to embrace it someday too!

CHAPTER 9

Medications Used for ADHD

HERE ARE SEVERAL PRESCRIPTION medications available for treating ADHD. Most of them are stimulants. Why do we give stimulants to a person or child who is already hyper? Researchers have found that when you give stimulants to people with ADHD, instead of speeding them up, the drug gets them on the right track. It's as if the brain shifts gears and the attention span increases, giving them more focusing ability. This is why it is a shame when parents won't at least try one of these drugs to see if it can help their suffering or struggling child.

The most commonly used stimulant is methylphenidate. It is found in an extended-release formulation in the following medications: Ritalin LA, Ritalin SR, Metadate ER, and Metadate CD.

More medications that are based on methylphenidate include the following:

- ☐ **Concerta:** *it differentiates itself from other methylphenidate pills because it has a special time-release technology.*

- ☐ **Daytrana:** *methylphenidate HCl in a transdermal patch. This differentiates itself from the others in that it is absorbed through the skin. This provides fewer side effects, and there is no pill to swallow. These patches have proven to be very long lasting, and the patient receives the medication very evenly throughout the course of the day.*

- ☐ **Focalin XR:** *another ADHD drug with dexmethylphenidate HCl. It is an extended-release capsule.*

Stimulants without methylphenidate include the following:

- ☐ **Adderall** *contains amphetamine and dextroamphetamine, and it comes in many different strengths. It also has an extended release.*

- ☐ **Vyvanse (lisdexamfetamine)** *is a newer formulation of an amphetamine.*

- ☐ **Nuvigil (armodafinil)** *is an alerting medication, which can help with ADHD symptoms. It was originally used to help with narcolepsy*

Nonstimulant medications include:

- ☐ **Strattera (atomoxetine HCl)** *is not a stimulant. Instead it is a norepinephrine reuptake inhibitor used to treat ADHD. It increases the norepinephrine and dopamine in the frontal cortex of the brain. This is very effective with many children, and it doesn't have the same side effects as stimulants.*

- ☐ **Intuniv (guanfacine)** *is another, newer nonstimulant drug with a smoother formulation of an old drug.*

Possible Side Effects of Stimulants

The most common side effects of stimulants are poor appetite (which can contribute to weight loss), irritability, trouble sleeping, excess crying, headaches, stomachaches, and anxiety. Some of these are symptoms that many kids with ADHD already portray without medication. That is why it is nice to have options when it comes to choosing a medication for your child. The doctor needs to take into consideration what is going on with the patient before prescribing a medication. Depending on the characteristics that your child may be displaying, a doctor can decide which medication will benefit your child the most. Another side effect that is not really common but can occur in children as well as adults is tics. Tics are small jerky movements that become repetitive when the medication is typically too strong. Usually once the medication is adjusted down the tics go away.

Persistent adverse side effects should not be tolerated! Here are Ten Principles of Treatment with Psychoactive Medications created by our specialist, Dr. Brutoco:

1. The goals of any psychopharmacologic intervention with any child or adolescent should include the promotion of more normal patterns of maturation and development.

2. The use of psychoactive medications should not be used as an "either/or" issue. Medication must be considered an integral component of a comprehensive therapy program.

3. Medication doses should generally be initially very low, then titrated to the particular needs of each individual patient. Medicine should be gradually increased until desired effects are achieved, and then continually adjusted until it is no longer deemed necessary and then very gradually weaned.

4. It is obvious that treatment with potentially powerful medications should facilitate real changes in the patient. In order to do so, the medication will have effects on various mental and physical systems and functions. These effects and functions must be regularly monitored throughout the course of treatment.

5. Effective monitoring requires an ongoing collaborative effort among patient, family, and physician. It is vitally important that there be regular, scheduled direct clinical contact, as well as input from patient/family to physician on both a regular basis and in the event of changes in the patient's condition/well-being.

6. If positive effects are noted, but stability is difficult to achieve with one medication, adding a second medication is often preferable to discontinuing or changing the primary medicine. Similarly, multiple meds working synergistically for a total beneficial effect is often reasonable and appropriate.

7. Individual variations are common, and a flexible, personalized approach to treatment must be maintained by both the physician and patient/family.

8. Once discontinued, careful clinical monitoring of performance, attitude, behavior and self-esteem should continue for an extended period.

9. Positive effects of treatment must not only merely outweigh negative effects but rather substantial and prolonged undesirable side effects must not be tolerated. Medication adjustments are indicated until positive results continue without medication-related problems of significance.

10. Reliable compliance with an uninterrupted treatment course is essential.

Antidepressants

Why are antidepressants sometimes prescribed with ADHD Medications? The reason some psychiatrists prescribe antidepressants with the ADHD medications is to alleviate the side effects of the methylphenidate. Antidepressants such as Zoloft (sertraline), Celexa (citalopram), Lexapro (escitalopram oxalate), Wellbutrin (bupropion), and Remeron (mirtazapine) help to take away the irritability, loss of appetite, and anxiety that can be brought on with the ADHD medications. Most of these drugs have been around for a very long time and are known to be safe and effective medications. All three of my children have been on many of these medications, and the greatest result my kids have had is that they do not suffer from the more severe side effects of the stimulant medications.

The greatest compliment I have received is that no one can believe that my children are medicated. The goal in medicating people and children with ADHD is to find a combination of medications that will most benefit them without them feeling or acting drugged.

As you read through this book you can see how many different medications my kids have taken. That is the greatest challenge with using medication to treat ADHD symptoms.

Everyone is different, so that is why there are so many medications out there to try, and the pharmaceutical companies are making more every year. These medications will be different with each person who takes them, and the side effects and success of the drug depend on each individual's weight, height, metabolism, personality, hormones, and sensitivity to certain chemicals. This process does require patience and you must keep trying until your child feels great. The results of the right medication are priceless!

CHAPTER 10

What a Difference Medication Makes

OUR FAMILY STORY COULD have had a much different ending if it hadn't been for medication. Over the years I have come across many parents with kids who had very similar symptoms to my children, but the parents felt that their kids were in a phase that they would outgrow so they never got them help. I have received many phone calls over the years from parents whose kids were Portlan's age and had suffered with symptoms of ADHD. Many of these parents we met through baseball, school or in our neighborhood and they could not believe the transformation Portlan made from age ten, when they saw him at his worst, to fifteen, when he was motivated, doing well in school, and was very involved in sports and the church youth group. These parents' kids were barely able to get out of high school. A few of them are now using drugs and living on the street. Some kids whom managed to graduate have no motivation to even get a job, let alone go to college. These were the same parents who believed their kids were just going through a rough patch and would grow out of it.

If you get anything out of this book, at least try to find help for your child through a psychiatrist or MD who is educated about ADHD if you think your child might have ADHD/ODD. They are very real disorders, and your child can't help his or her behavior and what he or she is doing. Don't be the parent who just goes into denial and waits for things to change. Our children need our help. As parents, that's what we are here for, and if we don't help them who will? Yes the doctors and medication can be expensive, but you can pay now with a chance at a positive outcome, or pay later.

Here is another disturbing statistic: one quarter of the men in our jail system have some form of ADHD. The book *ADD Kaleidoscope: The Many Facets of Adult Attention Deficit Disorder*, by Joan Andrews and Denise E. Davis, discusses what characteristics are carried from childhood on into adulthood as well as the consequences of undiagnosed and untreated ADHD. This book also gives examples of people who have three different societal backgrounds as well as their symptoms and how each person ended up in the jail system because of their uncontrolled impulsivity, tendency towards anger and rage, and the thrill of danger and fear that can drive their emotions and actions.

These disorders are not over diagnosed in society; if anything they are under diagnosed. The best way to look at it is if there are thirty-two children in a classroom of which thirty of them can follow the rules and get their work done but two cannot; how can that be over diagnosed? If two children from every class in a school can be helped through medication or behavior management, how much better would society be? Think back to your own childhood and think of the awful kid in your class who was always seeking attention in an obnoxious way. The class clown was probably another kid who was trying to cover up learning issues. I know when I was in high school there was a continuation school that was full of troubled kids who were often caught smoking cigarettes or marijuana and abusing alcohol. I personally have never smoked a cigarette or tried any illegal drugs. People used to tease me about how was I going to know if my kids were on anything because I never tried any drugs. Fortunately, there is mother's intuition and even if you have to cheat a little to have it you can change your child's life. Portlan said to me one time, "Mom I love the way you always know when something is bothering me." Thank God this boy wrote in a journal and I knew where he hid it!

God blesses us with many challenges in this life. It's how we choose to overcome them that counts. My greatest challenge in life has been helping my children and my spouse "successfully survive the waves of ADHD" and not letting it change who they want to be in life. My challenge has now transitioned into a purpose and a passion to help the countless other families out there who are struggling with these very real disorders. Fortunately, there are some wonderful medications today that can help children as well as adults to function normally. Like any other illness though, a proper diagnosis needs to be made and nine times out of ten it is going to take a parent to see the red flags and take some action. You need to act quickly though because the longer you let these symptoms go the harder they are to correct.

Attention Deficit Hyperactivity Disorder doesn't have to destroy a child or a marriage. Today's society expects so much more out of our children and it is our job as parents to prepare our children for these pressures and not let society crush them along the way. My intention for writing this book was to give readers HOPE and FAITH for their child's future. My hope being, that by reading my story of many challenges that turned into successes will provide the faith you need to feel confident in the difficult decisions that need to be made with your children through your families own waves of ADHD. It is when you accept your children for who they are that you really get to know who they are. You need to accept and embrace ADHD in your child because he or she is an exceptional individual. With the proper guidance your child can and will be extremely successful in life.

Selected Bibliography

Andrews, Joan, and Denise E. Davis. *A.D.D. Kaleidoscope: The Many Facets of Adult Attention Deficit Disorder.* Duarte, CA: Hope Press, 1997.

Dobson, James C. *The Strong-Willed Child: Birth through Adolescence.* Carol Stream, IL: Tyndale House, 1985.

Gurian, Michael. *The Wonder of Boys.* 10th ed. New York: Tarcher, 2006-09.

Hallowell, Edward M., and John J. Rately. *Driven to Distraction: Recognizing and Coping with Attention Deficit Disorder from Childhood through Adulthood.* New York: Simon and Schuster, 1995.

Pollock, William. *Real Boys.* New York: Henry Holt and Company, Inc., 1998.

Stimmel, Barry. *Alcoholism, Drug Addiction, and the Road to Recovery: Life on the Edge.* Binghamton, NY: The Haworth Medical Press, 2002.

Stock Kranowitz, Carol. *The Out-of-Sync Child.* New York: The Berkley Publishing Group, 1998.

About the
Author

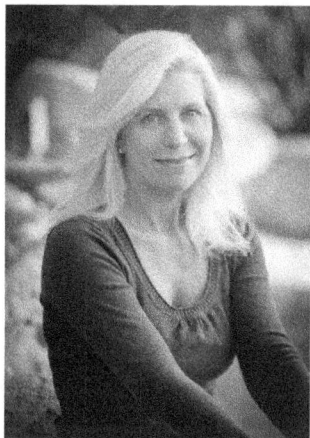

NANCI BECKMAN RESIDES IN Mission Viejo, California, with her husband, daughter, and three dogs. She plans to start speaking at local schools to help equip parents with a better understanding of Attention Deficit Hyperactivity Disorder. When talking with her you immediately experience her sense of humor and sincere belief that people need to understand ADHD and realize that it is not a one-time event nor is it an obstacle that can't be overcome. She continues to deal with the waves of ADHD with all of her children and spouse, making the most of her challenges.

www.surviveADHD.com